Blooming Bellamy

Blooming Bellamy

Herbs and Herbal Healing

David Bellamy

With Illustrations by Derek Hall

BBC BOOKS

ACKNOWLEDGEMENTS

Juliet S. Stoy and Gervais Productions for research, word-processing and preliminary edit.

This book is published to accompany the
television series entitled *Blooming Bellamy*.
The series was produced by
John Percival/Ark Productions for
BBC CE and Training Department, and was
first broadcast in Spring 1993

Published by BBC Books
a division of BBC Enterprises Ltd,
Woodlands, 80 Wood Lane,
London W12 0TT

First published 1993
© Botanical Enterprises (Publications) Ltd 1993
ISBN 0 563 36725 3
The moral rights of the author have been asserted

Illustrations by Derek Hall
© Derek Hall 1993

Set in 11/14½pt Monotype Baskerville by Selwood Systems, Midsomer Norton
Colour separation by Radstock Reproductions Ltd, Midsomer Norton
Printed and bound in Great Britain by Butler & Tanner Ltd, Frome
Jacket printed by Lawrence Allen Ltd, Weston-super-Mare

CONTENTS

TO R<u>OSE</u>MARY
Rosmarinus officinalis

'Comforteth the braine, the memorie, the inward senses ... the floures made up into plates with Sugar after the manner of Sugar Roset and eaten, comfort the heart, and make it merry, quicken the spirits and make them more lively.' So wrote Gerard of London in 1597.

On all that I can agree, for Rosemary Bellamy née Froy has been my constant companion in sickness and in health for almost forty years.

DAVID BELLAMY, BEDBURN 1993

Rosemary

(14) (Poison ××) Rosmarinus officinalis (5–7)

Rosmarinus means 'dew of the sea' and it is the plant which helps give that unforgettable fragrance to the shrublands which border the Mediterranean.
CONTAINS an essential oil rich in terpenes, cineol, borneol and pinene.
USES: decorative, flavouring, fragrance.
 C: cure-all, insecticide and an abortive.
 HER: carminative, digestive, rheumatism, ulcers, eczema, herbal baths.
 HOM: none. Today a mainstay of aromatherapy.

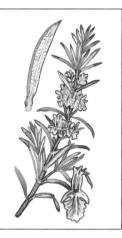

NOTE ON PLANT BOXES

The number in brackets after the common name is the number of prescriptions in which the plant was used by the Physicians of Myddfai (see page 30). The numbers in brackets after the Latin name are the numbers of the months during which the plant is in flower in Britain.

The following abbreviations occur in the plant boxes found in the main text of the book: *C* for uses in Classic Medicine, *HER* for uses in Herbal Medicine, *HOM* for uses in Homeopathic Medicine and *R* denotes the results of or uses in recent research.

It's an Ill Wind

'Get away, get away, get away for a day in the country', so goes the refrain of the music-hall song, and most townies, or urbanites as we now call them, try to do just that. Those cherished, invigorating, rejuvenating days of leisure, those breaths of fresh, unpolluted air.

But how pure is it? 'Find a spot by a shady lagoon and nature's waiting around to commune', and some of us find that oh so fresh air communicates in a rather vicious way, with its lethal bouquet of pollen grains replete with chemicals which make us sniff and snuffle, or much worse. For the luckier majority, these airborne natural impurities flow by unnoticed, indeed the very same passing fragrances – the tang of sea air, the smell of new-mown hay – add to our sense of well-being in the countryside. Apart from these essential oils and perfumes which tickle our fancies or inflame the innermost parts of our lungs, there are all those other things which can leak out from plants and evaporate into the air: alkaloids, anthracenosides, antibiotics, bitters, cardenolides, coumarin, flavonoids, glucides, heterosides, phenols, ranunculosides, resins, saponosides, tannins – and these are just a few of the many thousands of complex chemicals which may, as the temperature rises, season the air with their presence. Complex chemicals such as alkaloids could kill in large enough doses but in the minute doses released by the sun and atomised on to the wind might be a natural homeopathic cure-all which nature has put into place.

Since the advent of the motor car, people have been increasingly exposed to lead, especially in inner cities, lead which went unnoticed as a factor in human health until some very sophisticated statistics flushed it out. Likewise, the pollen count now given out with the daily weather forecast warns of the ill wind that blows asthmatics no good.

Could it be that if we only took the trouble to study air in the detail which it surely deserves we would also be able to identify the constituents in the healthful wind that blows everyone some good?

Modern research shows that insects can be turned on by just a few molecules of a chemical messenger called a pheromone which was released by a potential mate many miles downwind. Similarly, those sought-after fungi, the subterranean Truffles, contain chemicals which are certainly akin to pheromones produced by pigs and other mammals; while members of the plant family which includes the Mexican Yam produce chemicals which are very like our own sex hormones. It would therefore be ridiculous to dismiss the idea that complex creatures like humans, whose brains give us the power of conscious thought, cannot and do not respond to those chemical messengers which are all around us. We do know that our brains produce their own internal chemical messengers called endorphins. These are complex substances, very like the morphine produced by the Opium Poppy, which helps to take away all sense of pain from the body and mind and so aid the complex processes of recovery, healing and perhaps addiction.

Who knows? The research to prove or disprove the effects of natural chemicals in the air has never been done, yet over the centuries, nay the millennia since the dawn of human kind, kind human beings have done their best to cure the illnesses of their families and friends. Countrywide wisdom distilled over aeons of trials and errors has become part and parcel of the old wives' tales which passed down the knowledge of success through generations. Successful healing was rewarded with respect and recognition as a genial friend of the community; but too much success or failure was regarded with jealousy or mistrust and the result was the ducking-stool or worse. A country healer might be a midwife for all seasons or a witch for no reason at all.

My own apprenticeship with the healing power of plants was with Boots Cash Chemists at Cheam in Surrey where my dad was the manager and very proud of his certificate from the Pharmaceutical Society displayed on the wall. He translated the local doctors' scribble into copperplate records set down in giant leather-bound books; ancient knowledge made safer through the scruples of modern dosages.

If he got it wrong, the patient might die and he would have been to blame. I remember tinctures, two teaspoons to be taken before meals; inhalants and balsams dissolved in hot water and the vapours breathed in under a clean white linen towel (the linen itself made from the fibres of the Flax plant). Pills, their contents weighed with precision, coated with sugar, rolled out on a pill machine and polished in a round wooden tray made from the Common Box plant, which had also been used to make the ruler with which he slit the white paper to the exact size required. With deft hands he would then wrap the pillbox, packet or bottle, sealing the final flap with a drop of red sealing wax. I can still remember the aroma of the shop which he brought home with him, suffusing his clothes with the unmistakable heritage of *materia medica* (the raw materials of drugs mainly from plants).

My father was very proud of the modern medicines and as the new breakthroughs of the 1930s and 1940s came on-stream he would tell us about the way all the illnesses which had been the scourge of his young days were being conquered one by one. The first batches of commercial penicillin had to be dispensed under antiseptic conditions. This was accomplished by erecting a garden cloche in the dispensary with a nearby bunsen burner keeping the air moving upwards to carry would-be contamination away. Boils and carbuncles which to that time had been long and lingering afflictions painfully poulticed and drawn were suddenly things of the past now cured, or at least rapidly cleared up, by a waste product of a plant, a fungus called *Penicillium notatum*, originally found thanks to its spores having been blown in on the wind to Alexander Fleming's laboratory in St Mary's Hospital in London.

Dad was a pharmacist of the old school which meant having a firm grounding in Galenicals, healing materials from plants. Galen was a Greek physician born at Pergamum in Asia Minor around AD 130, he died in Italy some seventy years later and was the most highly respected physician of those times. His works on *materia medica* were the basis of medical study until the late seventeenth century and some of his recipes for healing were still being dispensed at Cheam in my childhood. Yet Dad was also steeped in the new and more complex traditions of patent medicine. The pharmacy's mahogany drawers which had once held leaves and roots, flowers, fruits and seeds now stored Dr Collis, Beecham's Pills, Owbridge's Lung Tonic, Linseed, Liquorice and Chlorodyne Lozenges, and Meloids. Even the ground-glass-topped jars and porcelain pots of the dispensary lost their Syrup of Squills, Elephants' toenails – sorry, Gum tragacanth and *Nux strychnos* which, thanks to the strychnine they contained, would kill anything except the dreaded but fascinating drug weevils – and belladonna which would do the same. These objects of fascination, which could be identified under the microscope as the bona fide BP article (BP stands for *British Pharmacopoeia*, the official reference book of all our chemists), were slowly replaced by white powders purified and compounded at the factory.

Thomas James Bellamy MPS was a staunch defender of the new and so, in his professional capacity, looked down upon those lesser establishments who, along with mops and brushes also made of plant material, still sold the ancient herbal remedies in their raw form. Yet he was part of the 'holistic practice' which had developed through time: a friend of all his customers, a knowledgeable intermediary between doctor and patient, part of whose job was to explain to his customers the whys and wherefores of the use of each and every new cure which came to hand. 'And make sure you finish the full course of treatment; don't give up half-way, however much good it's done you, you don't want it to start up all over again.' Wise counselling it would be called today; all part of that special relationship between healer and patient which has worked so well across the ages.

When my father retired he took up walking as a healthful hobby. Together, he and his best friend Frank Watkins, manager of the next branch of Boots, took to the mountains, hills and byways of Britain where they discovered in the natural vegetation many of the plants which had for so long formed the substance of their healing profession.

This book will allow you to follow in those footsteps and discover for yourselves the magical backdrop of our natural flora: a living carpet which once upon a time, and not that long ago, helped to order our lives season by season by producing a healthy dose of nature's own outdoor endorphins – healing chemicals in those healing draughts of fresh, country air.

Despite campaigning by many dedicated and well-informed people, our countryside has changed out of all recognition since I was a small boy. Ninety-seven per cent of all our flower-rich grasslands, more than 60 per cent of our lowland heaths and 50 per cent of what was then left of our ancient woodlands have been destroyed. The destruction included many plants which were and still are used in herbal medicine. We hear a lot about tropical rainforests and how they must be conserved, and the same is (equally) true of our own vegetation. Without the natural vegetation and the plants and animals which it supports and which support us, I believe the human race has little chance of survival. The fight is on! I hope that by reading this book and watching the television series that goes with it you will understand more of the importance of our own once common plants and join the fight to save them.

PS   Arguments have raged around herbalism, mainstream medicine and homeopathy since each was invented, or rather evolved, as people desperately tried to cure themselves and other people of various complaints, diseases and afflictions.

Herbalism is the most ancient form of medicine and many herbal cures have stood the test of time and are still present in modern medicines. What is more, over recent years even the largest pharmaceutical companies have once more begun to show great interest in the potential healing chemistry of the plant kingdom.

This book is **not** a do-it-yourself home doctor. Indeed, it is exactly the opposite and again and again issues firm warnings: medicine of whatever kind must only be practised and administered by highly qualified specialists.

All this book aims to do is to give you an insight into the wonder of some of the plants of Britain which have helped heal our landscapes and our increasing population over the past 12,000 years.

THREE IMPORTANT HEALTH WARNINGS

If you are unwell please go to see your doctor. Messing about with medicines on your own can cause grievous bodily harm or worse.

If your doctor decides to send you to a herbal or homeopathic practitioner, or if you decide yourself to go, please make sure that they have the full qualifications of their profession.

Also, in my young days I could pick a bunch of wild flowers for my mum's birthday and do no harm. Today this is no longer the case. Over the last forty years much of our natural vegetation has been destroyed. Please don't let this book tempt you to pick, dig up or damage any plant growing in the countryside.

CHAPTER ONE

We are what we eat

W̲e are what we eat and so, like the plants which are at the bottom of every garden and of every food chain, we are made of carbon, hydrogen, nitrogen, oxygen and an assortment of minerals. The first four we get from the atmosphere where they exist as invisible gases. Hands up all those who don't believe in ghosts! Well, over 99 per cent of each hand, and of all the rest of us, is made from the constituents of thin air, thanks, of course, to the plants. The last item, minerals, we and the plants get from the soil.

PLANTS AND ANIMALS

At some time in the dim and distant past, two groups of living things, bacteria and lowly little seaweeds, started to go their own complex ways. One group developed bodies mainly made of proteins; they became the 'move-abouters', the animals. The other group developed bodies mainly made of carbohydrate; they became the not-so-mobile plants. In time they became very different; the animals developed heads, bodies and legs, complete with skeletons, brains, blood, stomachs, livers and kidneys; the plants developed leaves, twigs, branches, trunks and roots, complete with a system of internal tubes and pipes for moving water, minerals and food from one part to another.

Animals and plants did, and still do, have an awful lot in common. Large plants and animals are made up of millions of tiny living units called cells which contain a jelly-like substance called protoplasm. This is full of minute yet complex structures, on and within which biochemical production lines function. These production lines are very similar in plants and animals. They all use energy and raw materials, and all produce waste, some of it very toxic. To deal with this, animals have complex internal systems focusing on the liver and kidneys, which detoxify the poisons and rid the body of them as quickly as possible. Plants are not so lucky; waste products produced in the shoots and roots have to be stored by the plant, out of harm's way. They are only got rid of when the leaves, stems, roots or bark drop off, or are eaten or collected by a passing animal.

FOOD CHAINS AND HEALTH STORES

In essence, and it is the essence of all life, plants make chemicals and animals either depend on these chemicals, develop an immunity to them or learn to leave them well alone.

Why exactly plants produce so many 'poisonous-to-life' chemicals we do not know but, if you can't run away from something that's going to eat you, then chemical warfare is perhaps the only way to grow and be successful.

We and all animals need carbohydrates, fats, amino acids (the building blocks of proteins) and roughage. Fortunately for us, these essential items make up the vast bulk of all plants and so of our diet. We in the rich First World know of the problems which come from eating too much of any of them, while many people in the poor Third World can't get sufficient for their needs and so die of malnutrition.

If we buy tins and packets of processed food we now expect to see them labelled not only with the nutritional value of the contents but also with a list of any chemicals which have been added during manufacture. We don't expect to receive that information with the fresh fruit and vegetables we buy but, if we did get it, we might be in for some nasty shocks.

Many of the most delicious and natural things we eat, even if they are grown under strictly organic conditions, contain a host of complex chemicals, some of which do us a lot of good and some of them capable of doing us a lot of harm.

Here is a breakdown of the things we need; we all know at least something about them thanks to stories on the back of the breakfast cereal packet.

VITAMINS

Vitamins are essential parts of the chemical production lines, hurrying the process along. Fortunately, plants need them too; they can make the most of them, we can't. All help promote normal healthy growth.

● **Vitamin A** is especially good for those membranes which keep us lubricated, healthy and growing. It also strengthens the eyes and helps us to see in darker places. Plants provide us with the orange-coloured raw material, our livers do the rest. The need for vitamin A is one reason why we add a little bit of parsley to so many dishes.

● **Vitamin B** – there are lots of B vitamins and we need them all. B_1 and B_2 tone up and help the working of our digestive and nervous systems. B_3 helps to keep the skin healthy. B_6 helps to digest your protein, and without B_{12} blood formation comes to a grinding halt. The best sources of the B vitamins are yeast and cereals, so cornflakes and real beer – both, of course, in moderation – can do you no harm and a lot of good. Moderation is the operative word for too much alcohol causes B_6 deficiency!

● **Vitamin C** aids the formation of bones, activates the transfer of energy within cells (and energy transfer is the essence of life), tones up the blood vessels and helps the body by preventing certain infections, even, some say, the dreaded and still common cold. One of the best sources is rose hips.

● **Vitamin D** is a bone-maker and tooth-strengthener. The plants don't help us much with this one. Sunlight and open air are necessary for its formation in our bodies but yeast also helps. Lack of vitamin D in children leads to the deforming disease of rickets.

● **Vitamin E,** a prime mover working on your muscles and sex glands, is another vitamin found in cereals and in 'greens' but only if cooked properly, when they are a joy to eat.

● **Vitamin F** is good for the skin and for the arterial system, helping with those cholesterol problems which have been so much in the news lately. It also helps to soothe burns. Sunflower seeds are a good source.

● **Vitamin K** could be called the 'Popeye' vitamin because the best source of it is Spinach. However, this is one vitamin which we can make, with the help of the bacteria which live in our intestines. The raw materials, however, come from fresh green vegetables. Its main action is to help the blood to clot after injury and it is used widely in surgery.

● **Vitamin P** and **PP** – a group of vitamins which appears essential to the functioning of the capillaries, the tiny vessels of the blood system. Also good for the maintenance of the skin, and the nervous and digestive systems.

MINERALS

Minerals do similar jobs to vitamins but they are not manufactured by plants or animals. Instead, they are just passed along the food chain ready to be recycled. Plants suffer from mineral deficiency diseases and so do we. Fortunately, all healthy plants contain minerals and some concentrate them ready for our use.

Horsetail, that noxious weed of the garden, contains silicon, the stuff that glass is made of and an important constituent of skin, tendons and the cornea of the eye.

Dwarf beans, apart from being a good source of amino acids, and some very toxic compounds if eaten raw, are a rich source of potassium. This is one of the most important constituents of the body fluids such as blood plasma.

Saltwort, which grows by the sea, is so rich in common salt – another key component of those body fluids – that you can taste it if you chew the stems.

ANTIBIOTICS

Antibiotics first came to our notice in the 1940s, thanks to the work of Alexander Fleming and the fungus *Penicillium*. Antibiotics kill, or at least inhibit the growth of, other organisms, especially the bacteria whose ancestors were doing well on Earth long before there were any plants and animals.

The fascinating thing is that the more scientists look, the more of these defence chemicals they find, antibiotics and allelochemicals (growth retarders), produced by a wide range of living things. One of our commonest weeds, the Mouse-eared Hawkweed, contains an antibiotic used to combat certain fevers, while the Common Daisy produces a growth retarder that will chill you to the marrow.

HETEROSIDES

Heterosides are special sorts of sugar joined to something else which often puts a chemical sting into their tails.

All living things need sulphur, for that's what holds proteins together, allowing them to do all the clever things they and we do. Mustard contains more than its fair share of sulphur stored away in some very 'tasty' and 'nasty' compounds.

● **Cyanides** are made from hydrogen cyanide or prussic acid, and some plants such as Apples tuck it away in their pips which taste, just like bitter almonds, of prussic acid. Don't worry though, it is only there in very small amounts so an apple a day still helps to keep the doctor away.

Simple **phenols** are bacteriostatic which means they can stop bacterial infections in their tracks and so are very useful to both plants and animals, including us. One of the most famous plants containing these simple phenols is the Wintergreen, a North American shrub, from which the oil of wintergreen you rub on your chest is produced. The same chemicals give root beer its pungent flavour.

● **Flavonoids** are more complex phenols and many of them are pigments; plants produce coloured chemicals which were used in the dying industry for thousands of years before people even knew what they were. We now know that rue, one of the cure-alls of Greek medicine, contains vitamin P which does your capillary blood system a lot of good; it was first shown to be a pigment only in 1842.

● **Hay-scented heterosides** contain sweet-smelling coumarin. Coumarins and their near neighbours are still being investigated. Some are beneficial, most are poisonous if taken in too large a dose. Melilot, a common plant of grassland, will produce some really novel heterosides if fermented. It has now been synthesised and is used in cases of heart attack.

● **Anthracenosides.** Coal is, of course, made of fossilised plant material and in 1832 it was discovered that a chemical very useful in the dying industry could be extracted from anthracite. It was called anthracene. Looking round the plant kingdom, many modern-day anthracenes were discovered, some with helpful properties, often purgative. One, which has long been used and is rapid in action with nasty side-effects, is found in the very common Sheep's Sorrel, often used to put a bite into avant-garde salads.

● **Tannins** appear to be toxic waste products stored by plants in the trunk and especially the bark which is eventually cast off. They are phenolic substances and therefore help stop infection of plants by bacteria. They also promote the clotting of blood in animals. The strange Hart's-Tongue Fern is a good source of tannin and has long been used to treat disorders of the spleen and liver.

● **Bitters.** Many plants taste bitter and so must deter animals from eating them. However, bitters, which are complex and little-understood compounds, have for centuries been used to stimulate the appetite in humans.

● **Soaps or saponosides**, the penultimate group of heterosides, are apt to get everything into a lather. They are related to hormones and have a number of different effects on the human body. Heartsease, the weed which was selected and bred to give us the garden Pansy, contains saponins, and a ptisane made from the whole plant is recommended for nursing mothers.

● **Hormones** are nature's own control chemicals which keep living things in some sort of balance and order. They are complex internal messengers which switch on and off certain living processes. Seeing the great differences between plants and animals, it may seem strange to realise that down at the hormone level the two groups are being found to have much in common. Many plants contain the steroids which are the building bricks of animal hormones; steroids such as cardenolides which affect the heart, and diosgenin which helps determine human sexuality. Though not a British plant, the Mexican Yam must be mentioned here for it has given the world its most important medicine, the oral contraceptive pill, increasingly essential in this over-populated world.

ESSENTIAL OILS

Essential oils are better known than the diverse heterosides because they are much easier to detect: they smell. They are, in the main, very volatile chemicals which distil off from plants into the air, even on warm days in winter. These plants provide us with spices and aromatic herbs and flavourings. They also provide a fantastic variety of medicaments: oil of menthol, eucalyptus, mint and bergamot, the last also used in all the famous perfumes and in Earl Grey tea. Although essential oils are attractive to humans, many act as defence mechanisms for the plants making them distasteful to animals. Once concentrated, they become components of the resins which exude from plants, blocking up and disinfecting holes and wounds.

MUCILAGES

How does a plant grow? Well, in part it is thanks to mucilages, slippery compounds which lubricate the whole business. Pectins are well-known to all jam-makers and, along with the other mucilages, they help to store water. Once in the intestine, they help coat the inner lining, reducing irritation. If given in large doses they absorb water, swell and act as gentle laxatives.

A most unlikely source of medicine is the gardener's nightmare, the deep-rooting Couch Grass, yet its underground rhizome (the bit you can never dig out) contains 10 per cent mucilage, a diuretic and an antibiotic.

ALKALOIDS

Last, but by no means least, are the nastiest of all the plant-produced chemicals. More than any of the others, they probably do deserve the name of toxic waste. They are produced mainly by broadleaved plants growing rapidly in habitats which are rich in nitrogen.

Nitrogen has always been a major problem to living things; too little and we die, too much and death is even more rapid. The atmosphere is 78 per cent nitrogen, a gas which thankfully is chemically inert. If we all suddenly developed the ability to absorb nitrogen from the atmosphere we should be dead in seconds. Throughout evolution, nature has relied on tiny bacteria and Blue-green Algae, both of which were around long before the plants and animals went their own inter-related ways, to make the nitrogen in the air available to all other living things. Either living alone or in special root nodules in certain plants, these bacteria and algae 'fix' the nitrogen and then pass what they don't need on to their environment. Fortunately, most of the compounds they produce are soluble in the rain and so get washed away. However, any plants growing in the vicinity may well take up more nitrogen than they can handle, storing it away as the dreaded glycosides: chemical compounds whose properties have been used by witches, wizards, elves, poisoners, wise women, shamans and doctors through the ages.

One of the most beautiful plants is Monkshood, a cottage garden favourite which loves to grow near the compost heap or in forgotten corners near the sheep pens or soakaways near old outside loos. Monkshood is Europe's most poisonous plant and second only on a world scale to the Himalayan Monkshood from Nepal. The poisons are deadly and act in several ways: they can enter the body through the skin; the smell can cause nausea; as can smoke from a plant burning on the bonfire. Handle this plant with care, for in the right hands it has given the world a local anaesthetic; and treatments for rheumatism, neuralgia and the worst disorders of the skin. In the wrong hands or badly applied, it can cause great damage, and rapid death.

A little of what you fancy does you good and this is certainly true for all those vitamins, minerals and even the antibiotics and sulphur-containing heterosides. But what about all those other chemicals, and many more which science hasn't even got around to naming yet? Many have been a regular part of our diet and that of our ancestors; surely they haven't just passed through 'unnoticed' by the living system?

We may not believe the story of the Greek king who was so frightened of being poisoned by one of his courtiers that he regularly took minute doses of all the poisons so that he would be immune to a large dose. The legend goes that when his kingdom was under terminal siege he tried to end his own life to avoid the consequences of defeat. None of the poisons worked; he had indeed accomplished his original aim.

However, most of us today accept the fact of immunisation whereby small doses of the 'toxin' which causes the disease are administered and the body reacts by building up its own defence mechanisms.

The daily flow of low-dose chemicals in our diet could be working in much the same way or stimulating other hidden reactions. If the chemicals are harmful we would sooner or later know by feeling ill but if they were helpful it would be much more difficult to ascertain their presence let alone their effectiveness.

Mrs Warren Davies, one of our modern herbalists, believes there is another dimension to the complex picture. In a lecture she gave in 1977, entitled 'The Theory and Practice of Herbalism', she said:

Every cell in the human body contains a series of balancing mechanisms of stimulation and relaxation, controlled by complex feedback mechanisms. These intricate balances require a constant supply of nutrients, lack of any one of which over a limited time can be compensated for via some secondary pathway, but over a long period will create a chronic condition which is sometimes irreversible, but which can usually be corrected even in seemingly hopeless conditions with the use of the correct balance of nutrients.

Her philosophy makes good sense, and she puts it into healing practice by long-term treatment of patients suffering from a number of diseases, including multiple sclerosis.

In our normal 'balanced' diet which has evolved over the centuries, all the nutrients from amino acids and vitamins to all those still hidden and as yet unknown chemicals are supplied in a form ready for uptake and use by the plants we eat. Get the balance right and the vital cycle of life in each of the cells which make up our bodies will continue to turn in the direction of health.

CHAPTER TWO

A walk through the woods
❧

*T*he problem is that over the past thousand and especially the last 250 years it has become less and less possible for the people of the British Isles to do just that. Today less than 1 per cent of our land is 'ancient woodland' and all of that exists in a highly modified state. Its continued existence is thanks mainly to conservation groups such as the County, Woodland and National Trusts, the Royal Society for the Protection of Birds, the Forestry Commission and the Nature Conservancy Council in its new trinity of guises, English Nature, Welsh Countryside Council and Scottish Heritage.

Thanks to them, we can still appreciate that a walk through the cool, quiet dampness of one of their woodland reserves is of therapeutic value. It is tempting to say that we find our real chemical roots there amongst the trees from which our early ancestors originally descended and amongst which our more recent ancestors lived and breathed for so long. Roots hold the fertile soil on to even the steepest slope, and mighty trunks support a canopy aloft which shades and shelters a three-dimensional inner space: space untouched by the square-form bric-à-brac of modern life, space in which nature still reigns supreme.

> I think that I shall never see
> A billboard lovely as a tree
> But if the billboards do not fall
> I'll never see a tree at all.

Studies are now revealing the truth within Ogden Nash's twentieth-century lament. Patients in hospitals, suffering from a whole range of complaints and conditions, have been shown to get better more quickly if their wards look out on sylvan green than when they overlook concrete. The tradition of locating convalescent homes in countryside, and especially in mountain woodland settings, is supported by mounting evidence of their success – and not just because of the non-polluted air in which they are or at least were situated.

British forests come – or rather came, and should be being replanted – in three main sorts: acid Oak-woods on poorer and impoverished soils, lowland mixed woodland on nutrient-rich lowland soils and Pine and Birch woodlands especially in the North and other upland regions.

ACID OAK-WOODS

Oak had many uses in the times when everything from ships to windmills and cathedral roofs depended on or were suspended from oaken timber. In mythology, it was the tree of the Gods, reaching up to Zeus of the Greeks or Jove of the Romans, a tree which could not be struck by lightning. So it became an important part of parable and all types of divination.

> If the Oak is out before the Ash
> 'Twill be a summer of wet and splash,
> But if the Ash is before the Oak
> 'Twill be a summer of fire and smoke.

A dry summer is ideal for a bit of slash-and-burn land clearance, opening up more land for agriculture. This process eventually banished Oak from many of its strongholds. The Druids, holy men of the Celtic people who moved north-west across what was then a heavily wooded Europe long before Julius Caesar, worshipped Oaks, and especially the strange semi-parasitic Mistletoe which grew from its branches.

Mistletoe was cut with a golden sickle at the end of each year to be hung in houses to ward off bad luck. It supposedly had the power to avert evil influence so it was used to frighten away witches and the Devil. Such pagan rites and rituals were Christianised with the belief that Jesus's cross was made of Mistletoe wood, from which time forth the Mistletoe tree grew only in its reduced, semi-parasitic form.

Classical literature tells us that the twin berries fell from Uranus who was castrated with a golden sickle by Saturn, son of Jupiter. Falling into the sea, they gave birth to Venus or, if you will, Aphrodite, the Goddess of Love. So, to this day, at Christmastide we kiss beneath the Mistletoe. Tradition has it that one berry should be removed with each kiss; tradition also has it that Mistletoe must never be used for decoration within a church.

The berries have long been used in medicine and are also especially prized as aphrodisiacs. Although no proof has been found for this, research is continuing into other reputed properties of the plant, in helping the circulation of the blood and in arresting the growth of tumours.

Mistletoe is mistakenly called an epiphyte, growing as it does not on the soil but on the branches and twigs of trees. It is, in reality, semi-parasitic, drawing mineral nourishment by tapping into the wood of the host tree; but also tapping into the energy of the sun through the chlorophyll in its leaves.

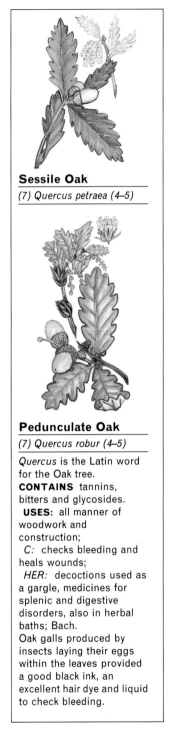

Sessile Oak

(7) Quercus petraea (4–5)

Pedunculate Oak

(7) Quercus robur (4–5)

Quercus is the Latin word for the Oak tree.
CONTAINS tannins, bitters and glycosides.
 USES: all manner of woodwork and construction;
 C: checks bleeding and heals wounds;
 HER: decoctions used as a gargle, medicines for splenic and digestive disorders, also in herbal baths; Bach.
Oak galls produced by insects laying their eggs within the leaves provided a good black ink, an excellent hair dye and liquid to check bleeding.

Mistletoe

(4) (Poison ××) Viscum album (2–4)

'Mistiltan' is an Old English word meaning 'different thing'.
CONTAINS mucilage, alkaloids and soaps;
USES: *C:* aphrodisiac, stitch and epilepsy;
HER: diuretic, heart tonic, for hypertension;
R: has shown that it acts by dilating the surface blood vessels, ongoing research into tumour therapy.

FERNS

The Oak-woods, especially those in deep shady gorges, overflow with an abundance of epiphytes and a great assortment of ferns. Ferns are vascular plants, which means their root and shoot systems are interconnected by an internal plumbing of microscopic tubes and pipes which transport water, minerals, sugars and internal chemical messengers from one part to another. The names Male Fern and Lady

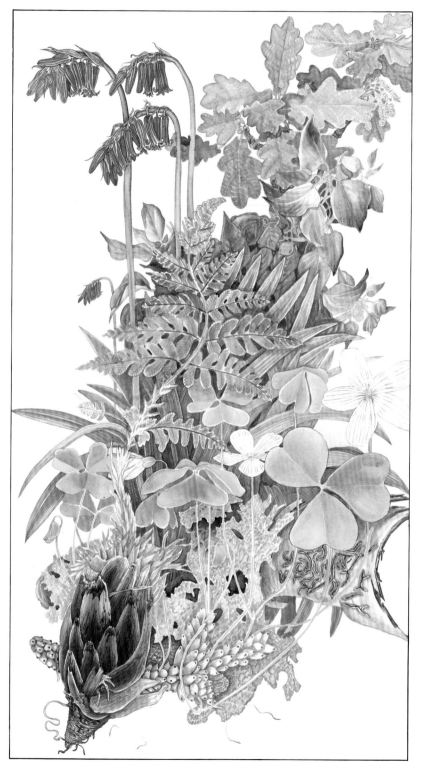

Pedunculate Oak Woodland on Acid Soils

1 Borrer's Male Fern, *Dryopteris borreri*
2 Wood Sorrel, *Oxalis acetosella*
3 English Bluebell, *Hyacinthoides non-scripta*
4 Sessile Oak, *Quercus robur*
5 Ivy, *Hedera helix*
6 Ancient Scribbler, *Graphis scripta*
7 Lungwort, *Lobaria pulmonaria*

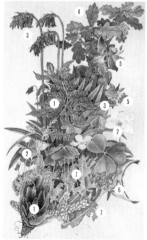

Fern have nothing to do with their sex, for all ferns are bisexual, the names simply refer to the plants' more robust and more delicate characteristics respectively.

Borrer's Male Fern (*Dryopteris borreri*) is a particularly handsome species with rust-brown scales covering the lower part of each main leafstalk and black blotches at the base of each main leaflet. Like many of our other ferns, it has been used for ridding humans and animals of intestinal worms. The worm-like roots

---

Borrer's Male Fern

(3) (Poison ×××) Dryopteris borreri

Borrer is the name of a famous botanist.
CONTAINS acids, essential oils and sugars;
USES: *C:* deworming, especially tapeworms;
 HER: rhizome used both powdered and as a decoction against internal worms;
 HOM: tincture, against ulcers, septic wounds and varicose veins;
 R: has shown that the worms are sent to sleep making them relax their grip on the wall of the intestine, a strong purge then gets rid of them and the poisons from the body.

---

which crowd its underground stem or rhizome and the black worm-like mass of the vascular tissue which appears when that organ is cut across perhaps led the herbalists to discover its worm-destroying properties. They saw the complaint depicted in the form of the plant and so, thanks to the idea of the 'Doctrine of Signatures' (see page 181), they discovered the cure.

EPIPHYTES

From our ferns to our epiphytes, those plants growing on another. The vast majority of epiphytes are mosses, liverworts, algae or lichens. One above all other British plants bears out the theory of the 'Doctrine of Signatures': its common name is Lungwort, in Latin *Lobaria pulmonaria*, and its shape and general texture is like a human lung dangling from the branches. In the hands of a herbalist these large thalli, for that is what the bodies of plants without definite roots and shoots should be called, yielded a soothing mucilage which would heal the sorest throat, chest and lung. Before the days when sulphur-rich coal took the place of wood as the main fuel for fire and furnace, large lichens like this were commonly found in woodlands, even around our largest cities. Then the lichens disappeared, killed off by rain polluted with sulphur dioxide, perhaps aided by over-collection by herbalists vainly trying to stem the upsurge of pulmonary complaints related to acid smog which, until the passing of the Clean Air Act in 1953, took its annual toll of lichens and people.

Another lichen which still abounds in the pure air of wetter western woods is *Graphis scripta*. If it had a common name it would probably be called the Ancient Scribbler for it runes its way along the twigs, its thallus erupting black through the thin protective bark. It must often have been included by mistake, along with other lichens, in many of the herbal medicines made from the bark of the tree, such as *Cortex Quercus*, a decoction used as a gargle, for bathing, and taken internally to treat disorders of the spleen and also enteritis.

Lichens are dual organisms, each made up of an alga (a distant relation of seaweeds) and a fungus. Take a close look at a lichen-covered rock, tree-trunk or even a gravestone and you will see how the discrete colonies of each species vie for all available space; some appear to get on well together, others to repel each other as if surrounded by a protective force-field. Thanks to the inspirational work of Alexander Fleming, our eyes have been opened to the fact that such force-fields do exist in nature in the form of antibiotics, chemicals emanating from the fungal component of the lichen. Exciting research is now discovering new antibiotics in lichens and in all sorts of unlikely creatures in the sea.

The Ancient Scribbler and its kin have been writing their own prescriptions of antibiotic success on the wooden walls of the forest ever since trees returned to these islands after the last Ice Age. Many lichens are fortunately still safe in those western wet Welsh and Scottish woodlands which, because of their high year-round water supply and humidity and their diversity of epiphytes and insects, well deserve the label of temperate rainforests and should be conserved along with all the other rainforests of the world.

The Ancient Scribbler links us to the people who first practised herbal medicine within our primeval forests, through the Physicians of Myddfai – pronounced Mudvi – a little village in south Wales. The strange symbols they used for weights and measures are not unlike some of the runes of *Graphis scripta* although some say they are more like Arabic script.

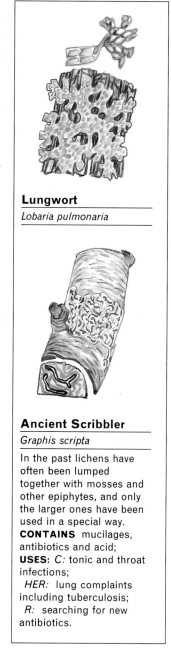

Lungwort
Lobaria pulmonaria

Ancient Scribbler
Graphis scripta

In the past lichens have often been lumped together with mosses and other epiphytes, and only the larger ones have been used in a special way.
CONTAINS mucilages, antibiotics and acid;
USES: *C:* tonic and throat infections;
HER: lung complaints including tuberculosis;
R: searching for new antibiotics.

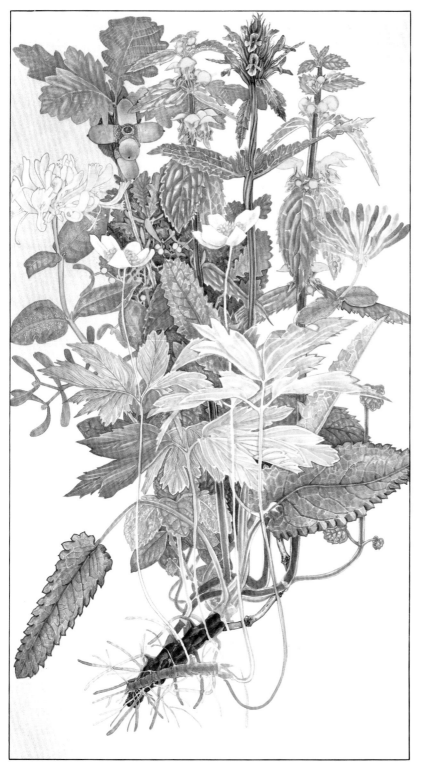

Sessile Oak Woodland

1 Wood Anemone, *Anemone nemorosa*
2 Wood Betony, *Betonica officinalis*
3 Mistletoe, *Viscum album*
4 Honeysuckle, *Lonicera periclymenum*
5 Sessile Oak, *Quercus robur*
6 Yellow Archangel, *Lamiastrum galeobdolon*

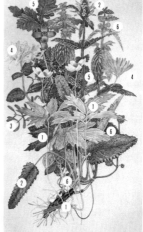

THE PHYSICIANS OF MYDDFAI

Despite all the legends and stories of the Lady of the Little Lake on the Black Mountain (see page 182), there is no getting away from the fact that a group of herbal doctors, probably all members of one family, served the Princes of south Wales in health and especially in sickness for about a thousand years. Some time in the twelfth or thirteenth century, one or more members of that group saw fit to ensure that at least part of their healing knowledge was passed on in the written as well as the spoken word. These ancient Welsh documents were first translated into English in the 1860s and published in the form of 815 prescriptions, recipes and recitals. Most of them refer to local plants which could, and still can, be gathered in that area of Wales. As such, they may well be the only written account we have of the body of Druidic herbal knowledge but other plants and concepts included in the writings also show knowledge of Greek, Roman and Arabic herbal and health practice and theory. Whether such knowledge came with the Druids as they travelled north or whether it was the result of later invasions or personal travel is not known. Nevertheless, the manuscripts are there, overflowing with food for holistic thought and worthy of much more modern research.

A walk through what is left of the woods around Myddfai brings you face to face with all the native plants used in the past. Two of the most conspicuous, thanks to their climbing and scrambling nature, are Ivy and Honeysuckle. The latter is in fact a true dangling plant better known as a Liana, one of only two found in Britain.

Ivy does not kill trees by strangulation as is popularly thought, its leafy presence may increase the likelihood of windthrow but, equally, its large woody twining stems prop up many a tree through its hollow old age. It is one of our last plants to flower each year, providing

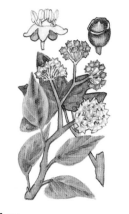

Ivy

(7) (Poison ×××) Hedera helix (9–11)

The berries can cause blistering of the skin.
CONTAINS soaps, glycosides, acids and resins.
USES: *C:* a panacea especially against the plague;
 HER: whooping cough, internal cramps;
 HOM: rickets, rhinitis and cataracts.

Ground Ivy

(18) Glechoma hederacea (3–5)

CONTAINS bitters, tannins and essential oils;
USES: brewing and clarification of ale;
 C/HER: digestive, tonic, ear drops for tinnitus;
 HOM: catarrh of the lungs, some types of asthma and intestinal infections.

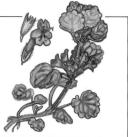

wasps and other insects, tempted out by sunny winter days, with both nectar and pollen. It provided the Myddfai with a novel way of extracting teeth, recipe 323:

> Take ivy gum and leaves, burn them into a powder in a new earthen pot, mix this powder with the juice of the herb petty spurge, and insert the paste in the tooth so as to fill the cavity. It will cause it to fall from your jaw, but have a care that it does not touch another tooth.

Dedicated to Bacchus, the God of Wine, Ivy was used both as an inn sign, signifying that wine was sold within, and as a morning after the night before cure for it was thought to prevent or relieve a hangover. Wine cups made from the Ivy wood were therefore highly prized by and in all locals. It was one of the first, and is still the most popular, of all house plants, cleaning the air in homes and offices across the world; an attribute of indoor plants now given the sign of approval thanks to research at no less a place than the American Space Research Institute, NASA.

Honeysuckle, the Liana, is on the other hand a very poisonous plant and ingestion should be avoided at all costs. However, and perhaps because of its tourniquet-like grip on the trees on which it grows, it was used both as an antidote to snake bites and as a contraceptive.

We come now to three plants which all bear the prefix wood to their common name. The first, a Sorrel, is thought to have been the original Shamrock of Ireland, the plant whose leaves St Patrick used to demonstrate the idea of the Trinity to the 'heathen' Celts. It was a good choice for, thanks to its sleeping leaves which fold up at dusk, it was already part of the Druidic Sun Wheel Cycle of belief.

The blush of pink on the frail petals of the Wood Anemone may have held special significance in the eyes of those who believed in the 'Doctrine of Signatures'; a flicker of

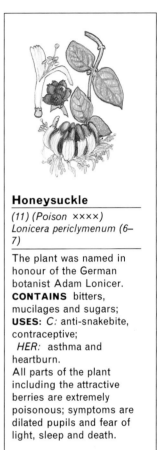

Honeysuckle

(11) (Poison ××××)
Lonicera periclymenum (6–7)

The plant was named in honour of the German botanist Adam Lonicer.
CONTAINS bitters, mucilages and sugars;
USES: *C:* anti-snakebite, contraceptive;
 HER: asthma and heartburn.
All parts of the plant including the attractive berries are extremely poisonous; symptoms are dilated pupils and fear of light, sleep and death.

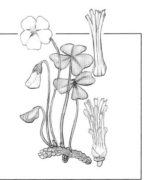

Wood Sorrel

(2) (Poison ××)
Oxalis acetosella (4–5)

Oxys is a Greek word meaning 'sharp' or 'acid'.
CONTAINS oxalic acid and bitters;
USES: removing iron stains from clothes, and cleaning brass;
 C: mouth ulcers and kidney complaints;
 HER: skin infections and cosmetic use.

life and therefore hope in the wan face of the sick. The plant was often worn as a talisman either around the neck or beneath the arm, where aroma-therapeutic uptake of the

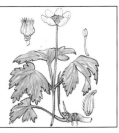

Wood Anemone

(Poison ×××) Anemone nemorosa (3–5)

Anemone is the Greek word for 'wind'.
CONTAINS ranunculosides, alkaloids and soaps.
USES: *C:* as a charm to keep away all diseases, especially leprosy and migraine;
  HOM: tincture for many things, almost a panacea.

chemicals it contains may have been helped by the warmth of the body.

Wood Betony is the plant no healer worth his or her salt would be without. It was used as a panacea, even curing hangovers; the tendrils of a Vine were said to turn away this witch plant rather than wrap it in their not-so-tender embrace. Nicholas Culpeper perhaps the best-known apothecary of all time (see page 184) wrote at length about this plant. He told his readers, 'It is a very precious herb, that is certain and most fitting to be kept in a man's house, both in syrup, conserve, oil, ointment and plaster.' Culpeper was in his own way an advanced thinker of his time. From his researches he knew that the healing power of the plants he used varied with time and even with the time of day at which they were collected, a fact borne out by modern research on plant physiology and biochemistry. The explanation he offered was that each plant was under the influence of the planets and affected by the moon and sun.

SIGNS OF THE TIMES

One plant which cannot be overlooked on any foray into our Oak-woods is the once ever-so-common Bluebell, although this should be called the English Bluebell, as Bluebell is the name given to the Harebell in Scotland. It has always been regarded as a plant of the fairies, something to be avoided. If picked by a child alone he or she would be lost, if picked by adults they would wander alone 'in and out the dusty Bluebells', until they felt the 'Tipper-ipper-apper on their shoulder' from the master who would lead them home – so chants the ancient play cycle. The sticky sap was used as a sort of starch for muslin and as a glue for papers and feathers but, as far as I can ascertain, not in medicine. The reasons for this are not clear; was it fear of the fairies or was the plant rarer back in the days of the

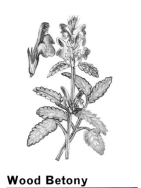

Wood Betony

(46) Betonica officinalis (6–9)

Gerard found a white form of the plant in a wood by a village called Hampstead, and took it into cultivation. He recommended a conserve made from the flowers for migraine.
CONTAINS tannins and acids;
USES: *C:* cure-all;
  HER: insomnia, varicose veins and sores;
  HOM: diarrhoea.

Physicians of Myddfai? Despite the fact that the flowers are today both common and especially abundant on poor thin acid soils, the great drifts we see are perhaps a more recent phenomenon linked to mismanagement and acid rain.

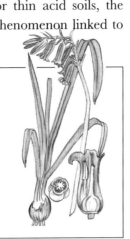

English Bluebell

(Poison ××)
Hyacinthoides non-scripta (4–6)

CONTAINS glycosides and mucilages.
The Bluebell does not grow naturally in central and southern Europe and so was neither named nor mentioned in the classical literature. This is probably the reason why it has been overlooked by medicine. All we can do is wonder why our own herbalists did not investigate the plant and what hidden virtues wait within.

IMPOVERISHED OAK WOODLAND

The general impoverishment of the Oak-wood soil from mis-management has led to increased acidity and a number of other major changes in the make-up of the vegetation. Birch trees have become more abundant and so has Rowan. The former is a tree of the upland forests, the latter pops up in most types of woodland and appears to thrive on disturbance. Rowan has always been looked upon as one of the great protective plants healing the landscape and protecting people against all sorts of evils, both imaginary and medical. Rowan wood was therefore incorporated into everything from the rockers of babies' cradles to make them safe, through pins to hold the ploughs firm on the shaft, to roof beams of barns and mighty houses. The fruits, which are not berries (which by definition have many seeds) but drupes are nevertheless full of vitamin C and make very good jellies and jams, protecting us against scurvy.

Another plant which appears to thrive under continued mis-management of our woodlands is the Foxglove. It has long been known by this name, as is proven by a mention of *Foxes glofa* in a plant list compiled in the reign of Edward III in the fourteenth century. Despite that, it was not a common plant in medieval gardens. Turner, one of the fathers of English botany, writing two centuries

Downy Birch

(2) (Poison ×) Betula pubescens (4–5)

Betula is the Latin word for the 'Birch'. Whole Birch trees were placed in farmyards and decorated with red and white cloths on Midsummer's day to keep witches away. As late as the reign of Edward IV in the fifteenth century branches were specially imported into London for the same purpose.
CONTAINS soaps, tannins, glycosides, resins and essential oils; the latter especially in the strongly scented variety found mainly in our uplands.
USES: wine making;
 C: magical rites and ceremonies;
 HER: diuretic, heart tonic, cosmetics, and the buds to stimulate digestion.

later in the reign of Queen Mary I, states, 'There is a herb that groweth very much in Englande and especially about Norfolke about the conie [rabbit] holes and in divers woddes [woods], which is called in English Foxglove.'

Its use in herbal medicine is recorded in the Myddfai prescription 274:

Take a handful of the leaves of foxglove, and a handful of the leaves of red nettles, pound them well, then boil in a quart of good honey, strain carefully and keep in a vessel. Boil therewith three pennyworth of the blessed water [of Rulandus], or distilled wine [brandy], or cider; then take two gallons of stale urine, boiling it well, and skimming it carefully as it boils. Take a quantity night and morning, and anoint your joints well therewith by the fire, rub them afterwards with the preserved ointment, rest your shoulder on an elevated place, and exercise yourself in walking frequently. It is good.

This was recommended for paralysis or hemiplegia, when the blood becomes sluggish in the veins. One can only hope that they got the dosage right, for Foxglove contains a deadly poison.

Some 400 years later, William Withering, a young doctor fresh out of the prestigious medical school of Edinburgh, was searching in vain for a cure for dropsy, a painful condition caused by bad circulation. One of his first patients was a young lady whose hobby was painting wild flowers. He fell in love with and later married her and so came face to face with the healing power of plants. Discovering that Foxgloves were used by the old wife herbalists of Shropshire, not far even on horseback from the Myddfai heartlands, he set about extensive experimentation.

He discovered, as herbalists such as Culpeper had done before him, that the amount of the active element present in the plant varied with its development; so detailed knowledge of the plant and

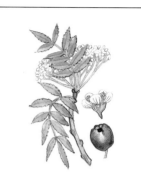

Rowan

Sorbus aucuparia (5–6)

A member of the Rose Flower Family. *Sorbus* is Latin for 'fruit'; *aucuparia* for 'catching birds', as the fruits are used as bird bait.
CONTAINS vitamin C, acids, the special sugar sorbose and acids;
USES: jams, jellies and preserves;
 C/HER: autumn tonic;
 R: sorbose is a safe sweetener for diabetics and is also used to reduce pressure in the eyes in glaucoma.

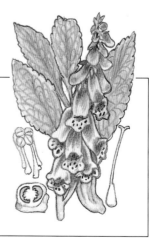

Foxglove

(10) (Poison ×××××)
Digitalis purpurea (6–10)

Digitalis is the Latin word for 'finger'.
CONTAINS several glycosides which include digitalin and digitoxine and soaps;
USES: *C:* dropsy;
 HER: heart tonic and dropsy;
 R: has shown that digitalin acts exclusively on the muscles of the heart.

its growth patterns was a prerequisite for making a preparation which contained a non-lethal dose. No mumbo-jumbo, no more relying on the phases of the moon or the apposition of the planets but instead pure science backed, unfortunately some would say, by the first use of animals in medical research. Up to that time all medicines and techniques (which included massive blood-letting, purging and treatment with compounds containing horrendous poisons such as mercury, arsenic and antimony), were tried out on the 'patients', perhaps even suggesting the derivation of that particular word.

William Withering, for better or for worse, made a great breakthrough in medical science using turkeys as his experimental animals. He realised that one could not summarily dismiss ancient instructions such as 'Gather only with the left hand from the north side of a hedge'. For an ultra-poisonous plant which should be handled with care, whose active elements increased in concentration as the flower spike slowly grew, and the slower the better, such seemingly frivolous instructions made good sense. From 1775 onwards the active element of the Foxglove, digitalin, became a standard and in many cases successful treatment for dropsy and a number of other complaints emanating from the heart. Only in very recent times has it been superseded by synthetic drugs and by open-heart surgery and transplants.

THE FLY AGARIC

Another plant which should be handled with care is the archetypal toadstool of children's books; you know, the one with a bright red cap and large creamy-white spots. The word toadstool comes from the German *todsthul* which means 'the stool of death' and the Fly Agaric, for that is its real name, should be left well alone. I would also make a plea that all fungi should be left alone for their own sakes and for ours. Please don't be frightened of them and knock them down, for left on their own they help to perform a very important job. Fungi are key components of nature's own clean-up gang which includes bacteria, insects and other animals; together they decompose and recycle all organic waste.

During the process of decomposition the fungi have to deal with all

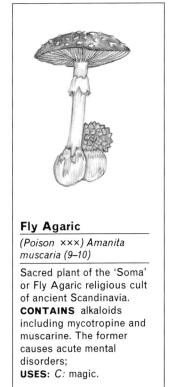

Fly Agaric

(Poison ×××) Amanita muscaria (9–10)

Sacred plant of the 'Soma' or Fly Agaric religious cult of ancient Scandinavia. **CONTAINS** alkaloids including mycotropine and muscarine. The former causes acute mental disorders; **USES**: *C:* magic.

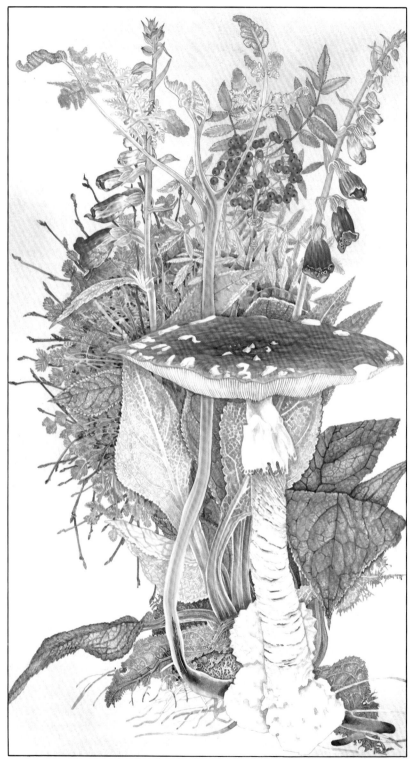

Impoverished Oak/Birch Woodland

1 Downy Birch (Witches' Broom), *Betula pubescens*
2 Foxglove, *Digitalis purpurea*
3 Bracken, *Pteridium aquilinum*
4 Rowan, *Sorbus aucuparia*
5 Fly Agaric, *Amanita muscaria*

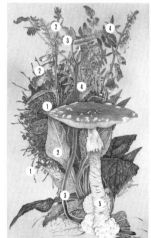

sorts of chemicals, many of them highly toxic, which are produced by the plants. Toxic waste dumps are not a new phenomenon and although all the natural products are biodegradable, something has to biodegrade them and it is little wonder that other toxic nasties turn up en route.

Like the red and black spots of our ladybirds, the red and creamy-white cap of this toadstool warns would-be predators, browsers or wily practitioners of the poisons or potions that lurk within. After much lethal trial and error, the people of the far north, who had fewer plants in which to seek their medicines, found a hallucinogenic drug within this toadstool. The drug had a unique property, for not only did it produce the desired effects, but it passed unchanged through the patient to be voided in urine whereupon it could be used again without fear of an overdose, although how they discovered this novel way of recycling we can only guess. The fame of this singular plant spread far and wide and is thought to form the origin of the fabled and sacred Soma plant of the Vedic medical tradition of India.

BRACKEN

Staying with the poison clan we come to another plant, Bracken. Today it is the most abundant fern found in Britain but when these islands were covered in forest it was, in all probability, much rarer and grew tall amongst the bushes in more open forest glades, searching for light. As the forest was slashed and burnt to make way for crops and grazing animals, the soil became impoverished and acid and Bracken came out of hiding and began its march across the open hillsides. One reason for its survival is that its shoots are charged with a fricassee of poisons including cyanide and carcinogens. The plants are therefore avoided by grazing and browsing animals including sheep and insects, sensible things that they are. Bracken has only one real enemy and that is frost, so it has rampaged across the country swallowing up farmers' lands and livelihoods. Little wonder that its spores, which on a warm summer night can cloud the air, are thought to allow you to disappear.

Unlike all our other ferns, Bracken spore masses are hard to see while on the plant because they are hidden beneath the folded edges of the leaves. So it was thought that Bracken produced its spores only on the Eve of St John, and that anyone who had possession of this magical and illusive powder could make themselves invisible. Despite its poisonous content and magical connections, the underground stem or rhizome was, and still is in places across the world, used as a food during famine. It is dried and ground then added as a non-nutritious flour in the making of bread. Other uses for Bracken have been found in the manufacture of soaps and detergents and in diet drinks and medicine; and modern research is again looking at this very common plant.

One piece of research you might like to try for yourselves, for it can do no harm if you are careful, is to cut one of the fronds where it is thickest below ground level. Look at the cut end of the stalk and there you will see, depending on your creed or kind, the initials of Christ, King John's Oak tree or the two-headed imperial eagle of Austria. The last gives Bracken its specific name *aquilinum*, meaning eagle.

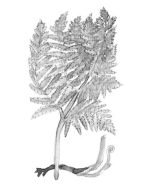

Bracken

(Poison ××××) Pteridium aquilinum

'Bracken' comes from the Anglo-Saxon word 'brake' meaning uncultivated land. **CONTAINS** salts of cyanide, glycosides, carcinogens and sugars. **USES:** *C:* famine food, magic, dressings for sprained joints, juice as eyedrops and for toothache.

MIXED WOODLANDS ON RICHER SOILS

Moving on from Oak-woods on acid soils to mixed woodlands on the richer soils, the palette of natural cures is found spread through no less than five main types.

Beech, though a native of the southern counties, has been planted far and wide across the length, breadth and altitude of the country. Beech leaves collected in the autumn were once used to stuff mattresses, giving them a tea-like fragrance which lasted for six or seven years and was said to help you to sleep. The leaves were also used for animal bedding and over-collection in the woodlands of Bavaria during the Second World War broke the natural recycling of nutrients, causing

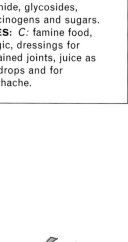

Beech

Fagus sylvatica (4–5)

Fagus is the Latin word for this tree and *sylvatica* means simply 'growing in the woods'. **CONTAINS** tannins, resins and alkaloids; **USES:** furniture making, creosote is distilled from the dry wood, and an edible oil is extracted from the seeds;
   C: water collected from the crotches of the large trees was used to clear up sores and eczema;
   HER: poultices, healing bruises.

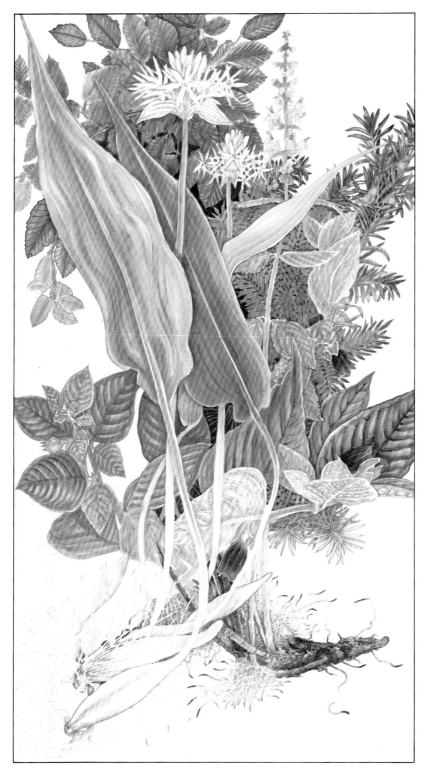

Mixed Woodland on Richer Soils

1 Wild Garlic, *Allium ursinum*
2 Deadly Nightshade, *Atropa belladonna*
3 Beech, *Fagus sylvatica*
4 Wood Sage, *Teucrium scorodonia*
5 Yew, *Taxus baccata*

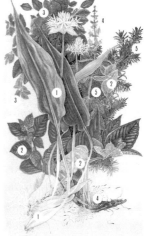

a marked increase in the acidity of the soils and loss of numerous lime-loving plants from the ground flora. Beechmast is another name for the fruits which, in a good or mast year – reputedly one in seven, was an important food source for wild and domestic pigs. Another name for the mast is buck, and this is where Buckinghamshire which is famous for its Beeches gets its name.

The dense leafy canopy created by Beeches prevents the development of a diverse ground flora. However, autumn brings a rich reward of toadstools and other fungi, and in the more open patches Wood Sage, Wild Garlic and even Deadly Nightshade may be found. The last is a member of the plant family which provides us with such useful foods as Potatoes and Tomatoes, which were originally brought to Europe from South and Central America.

The deadly nature of the Nightshade is encapsulated in its Latin name *Atropa belladonna*. *Atropos* was one of the Three Fates who wielded the shears which cut the thread of life of everyone, regardless of class or kind; *belladonna* means beautiful lady, and atropine, one of the plant's active elements, was used to dilate the pupils and widen the eyes while at the same time blurring the vision of ladies. It was still used for this reason when I was young by doctors prior to eye examinations. The plant was also linked with Hecate, Goddess of the Underworld, who knew the names of all plants and taught their uses and their virtues to her daughters: a liberated version of the Myddfai legend.

The Nightshades are close relatives of the much more infamous Mandrake, whose roots often take on human form. It does not grow wild in this country but can be cultivated. The scream of a Mandrake when being pulled out of the earth was thought to be so terrible that

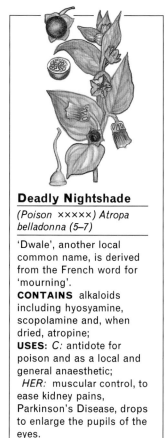

Deadly Nightshade

(Poison ×××××) Atropa belladonna (5–7)

'Dwale', another local common name, is derived from the French word for 'mourning'.
CONTAINS alkaloids including hyosyamine, scopolamine and, when dried, atropine;
USES: *C:* antidote for poison and as a local and general anaesthetic;
  HER: muscular control, to ease kidney pains, Parkinson's Disease, drops to enlarge the pupils of the eyes.

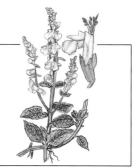

Wood Sage

(1) Teucrium scorodonia (7–9)

CONTAINS essential oils, tannins and bitters;
USES: *C:* bitter tonic and digestive, prevents flatulence, against venereal diseases, and for cleaning teeth;
  HER: healing wounds, rheumatism.

it would kill a man or woman, so a dog was tied to the plant and left to do the job out of earshot of its owner. Similarly, when gathering Nightshade, a black hen had to be let loose to lure away the Devil. Both the apple of

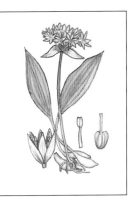

Wild Garlic

(1) Allium ursinum (4–6)

CONTAINS essential oils, glycosides with sulphur, vitamin C;
USES: as a culinary herb until true Garlic, which had been raised to the level of a God by the Egyptians, was introduced from the Mediterranean;
HER: internal and external antiseptic, ridding the body of parasitic worms, also of use against amoebic dysentery and flatulence;
R: shows Garlic helps in the reduction of fever and against the hardening of the arteries.

Mandrake and the black berry of the Deadly Nightshade were used both as local and general anaesthetics, often one supposes with disastrous results blamed on the Devil not upon the dosage.

Wood Sage was widely used until it was replaced by the tall blue garden Sage from Central Europe, which was grown both as a pot and a medicinal herb. An ancient Arabic saying counsels, 'How shall a man die who hath Sage in his garden'; while plantswoman and garden designer Gertrude Jekyll suggested that our own less showy plant deserved its place in the herbaceous border, and she should know being famous for such borders. Sage makes an excellent ground-cover plant and infuses the garden with goodness.

Our own Wild Garlic was also used for culinary and medicinal purposes until it too was replaced by the larger more rumbustious plant from the Mediterranean and beyond. It has a long history: it was raised to the level of a god by the Egyptians and consumed in vast amounts during the building of the pyramids. Garlic cultivation became part of the home front effort of the First World War and was commonly used as an antiseptic in the trenches before fungal antibiotics had been discovered or, to be more exact, rediscovered by modern medicine as there is written evidence that they were also used by the Egyptians.

Garlic Mustard, now a common plant of roadside verges, is also known as 'All Sauce' as it makes a good allround condiment. Much research still goes on to discover all the true virtues of the Mustards we use. English Mustard is best made fresh with cold water; our body temperature then stimulates chemical reactions which release some of its special properties. If made with water over 45°C (113°F) other

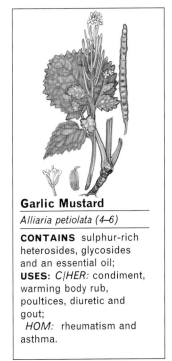

Garlic Mustard

Alliaria petiolata (4–6)

CONTAINS sulphur-rich heterosides, glycosides and an essential oil;
USES: *C/HER:* condiment, warming body rub, poultices, diuretic and gout;
HOM: rheumatism and asthma.

Lesser Celandine

(1) (Poison ×××) Ranunculus ficaria (3–5)

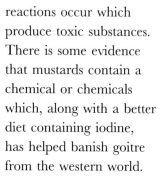

Rana is the Latin word for 'frog', and the plants bearing this name also live in damp places.
CONTAINS ranunculosides, soaps and flavones;
USES: *C:* the plant was carried with the heart of a mole as a talisman against enemies and lawsuits. The roots, which bear some resemblance to the udders of a cow, were hung in the byre to aid milk production; they also look like piles so were used to treat that affliction. Also used against warts, jaundice and for whitening teeth;
  HER: skin problems and bronchitis.

---

reactions occur which produce toxic substances. There is some evidence that mustards contain a chemical or chemicals which, along with a better diet containing iodine, has helped banish goitre from the western world.

Purging Buckthorn

(Poison ×××) Rhamnus catharticus (5–6)

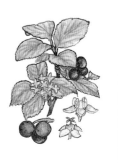

A Christian symbol of martyrdom, thought to be the plant that made the crown of thorns used at Jesus' crucifixion.
CONTAINS glycosides, resins and pigments;
USES: *C:* to ward off evil;
  HER: purgative, diuretic, blood purifier. This was one of the classic, or should the word be catastrophic, Victorian purges. It gives the patient an intolerable thirst.

Lesser Celandine is a common plant of woodlands and streamsides throughout the British Isles, in Orkney it is thought to have been introduced as a medicinal plant. Extracts of the root tubers, which look not unlike a bad dose of piles, have been long used to treat that affliction. A member of the Buttercup Family, it is not related to the Greater Celandine which is a relative of the Poppies.

Purging Buckthorn is a shrub or small tree which appears to like its roots in damp calcareous soil. Its fruits which turn from green to black provide a number of dyes and a very strong purgative. So strong that Gerard described how the berries were meted out by number, strong bodies taking fifteen to twenty. He called it Laxative Ram and so it was used until its place was taken by Casara sagrada – Spanish for Holy Bark, from another tree from the same family the Rhamnaceae.

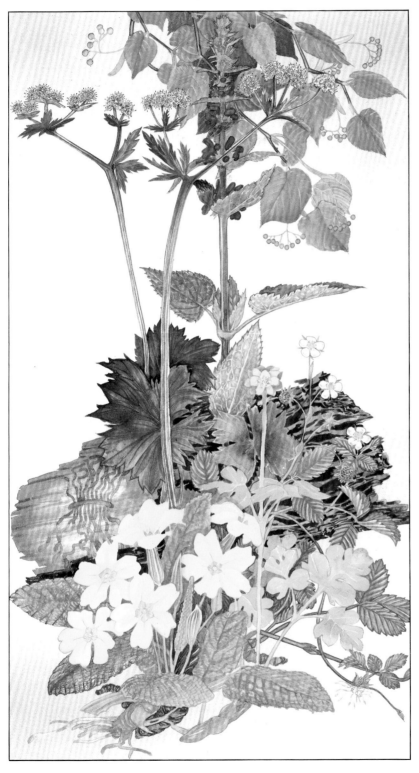

Elm/Ash Woods

1 Primrose, *Primula vulgaris*
2 Elm, *Ulmus procera*
3 Sanicle, *Sanicula europaea*
4 Small-leaved Lime, *Tilia cordata*
5 Hedge Woundwort, *Stachys sylvatica*
6 Moschatel, *Adoxa moschatellina*
7 Wild Strawberry, *Fragaria vesca*

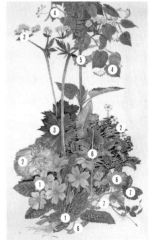

LIME AND HORNBEAM WOODS

In the warmer drier south, Hornbeam and Small-leaved Lime once dominated the sylvan scene. The latter is probably our only native Lime or Linden, its broadleaved counterpart and their hybrid being the result of introduction.

To sit beneath a Lime in June when it is in full flower is a never-to-be-forgotten experience, for the buzz of insects by day and the almost heady fragrance by night highlight the symphony of chemicals distilled into the air. One word of warning, never park your car beneath a Lime for aphids' droppings, otherwise known as honeydew, can mutate your turtle-wax job into a spotty monstrosity. Before the days of the automobile, but not that long before, the Lime was regarded as the 'life index tree' to the family upon whose land it stood; for example, a fallen bough foretold death in the family. The Lime tree which has greatest claim to botanical fame is the family tree which, in the late seventeenth century, stood in front of a small farm

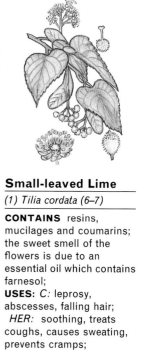

Small-leaved Lime

(1) Tilia cordata (6–7)

CONTAINS resins, mucilages and coumarins; the sweet smell of the flowers is due to an essential oil which contains farnesol;
USES: *C:* leprosy, abscesses, falling hair;
 HER: soothing, treats coughs, causes sweating, prevents cramps;
 R: the soft tissue or bast taken from beneath the bark is said to be good for rheumatism.

Primrose

(7) Primula vulgaris (12–5)

My mother was born on 19 April, Primrose Day, so it is another favourite plant of mine. Once so common, even around London, that I could pick a bunch for her birthday, sadly this is no longer so. But if we all care enough, we can put the Primroses and all our other wild flowers back where they belong. Children used to eat Primrose flowers, believing they would see fairies.
CONTAINS soaps, acids, glycosides, flavones and aspirin-like chemicals.
USES: *C/HER:* whooping cough, bronchitis and pneumonia;
 HOM: a tincture for neuralgia and kidney complaints.

Moschatel

Adoxa moschatellina (4–5)

Adoxa comes from the Greek word for inconspicuousness. To find this tiny plant with its five clock-like flowers looking in all directions but down always makes me feel good and that's why I have included it. When damp, as it usually is, the whole plant produces a faint but unmistakable smell of musk.

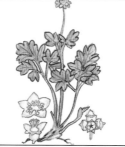

in Smäland in Sweden. It gave the family name of Linne to the son of the household, Carl Linnaeus, who in turn gave the world of science the (binomial) method of giving all living things two Latin names. Correct identification and naming using an internationally understood system is today a cornerstone of all herbal science. So next time you take a Lime tea, raise your cup to Carl Linnaeus and make sure you have picked the flowers yourself from your own tree and dried them in bunches in the sun.

The presence of the Small-leaved Lime indicates you are probably standing on the site of ancient woodland, much of which was unfortunately lost in the Second World War when the Lime-scented timber was used in the construction of Mosquitoes, aeroplanes with two stings in their tail.

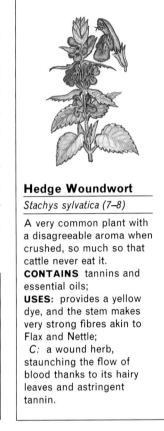

Hedge Woundwort

Stachys sylvatica (7–8)

A very common plant with a disagreeable aroma when crushed, so much so that cattle never eat it.
CONTAINS tannins and essential oils;
USES: provides a yellow dye, and the stem makes very strong fibres akin to Flax and Nettle;
 C: a wound herb, staunching the flow of blood thanks to its hairy leaves and astringent tannin.

Sanicle

Sanicula europaea (5–7)

The word sanicle probably comes from St Nicholas, one of the earliest medical saints. This is the only common name it has.
CONTAINS soaps, tannins and bitters;
USES: *C/HER:* one of the great wound herbs for both internal and external use, but not for wounds on the head.

As the woodland disappeared so too did the habitat for some of our commonest woodland plants such as Sanicle, Primrose, Wild Strawberry, Hedge Woundwort and Moschatel. All these fortunately found some sanctuary along our hedgebanks and disused railway lines, the latter being one definite benefit of the post-Beeching era.

ELM AND ASH WOODS

Elm and Ash take over on the damper heavier soils, and the more open, almost feathery canopy of the Ash provides light in plenty down at ground level so promoting a rich and varied flora.

Ash or Yggdrasil was the tree of life for the Vikings. They used its magical timber to construct the boats in which they came to Britain, bringing with them the vices and virtues they had found in sacred and in healing plants. Their beliefs included: a child suffering from rickets or a hernia could be cured if passed through a split Ash sapling; a leaf with an even number of leaflets placed under a maiden's pillow would reveal her future husband; a lock of the patient's hair fixed to an Ash tree would cure whooping cough. Perhaps the strangest cure of all was to send a bed-wetter out to seek and select an Ash tree. The next day he or she was sent to collect the fruits, or keys, from that same tree with their left hand and carry them home in the hollow under their right arm. Once home, the keys were burned on the hearth and after urinating on the ashes the person was cured. Could it be that homeopathic doses of fraxin, one of the active elements of Ash, safe in the warmth of the armpit, suffused in through the skin? Fraxin is a powerful diuretic and to this day Ash leaves are used in the treatment of rheumatism, to help the flow of urine cleanse the body, the natural way.

In Scotland we find the virtues of yet another herb administered in the same way. It is St John's Wort, called in Gaelic *Achlasan Chaluimchillo*, which translates as 'St Columba's armpit-package', and a packet of the herb was placed under the armpit of the patient to help internal healing.

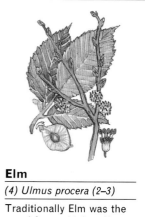

Elm

(4) Ulmus procera (2–3)

Traditionally Elm was the wood from which coffins were made, both ready for recycling, the final cure. **CONTAINS** tannins, mucilages and bitters; **USES:** *C/HER:* wounds, gout, skin diseases and burns; Bach.

St John's Wort

(4) Hypericum perforatum (6–9)

Was it the glands on the leaves, which make them look perforated with tiny holes, or the oily red juice which comes from both stems and flowers which made this one of the best-loved herbal remedies of classical times? Whatever the answer, right across Europe on the Eve of St John (two days after the summer solstice) fires were lit and this plant which had been collected in the morning dew was further sanctified in the smoke. It was used as a cure-all, a panacea against all evils and all ills. One word of warning, when taken to North America under the name Klamath Weed, it soon ran out of control and sensitised the skin of white cattle to the sun.
CONTAINS glycosides, oils and pigments;
USES: *C:* cure-all, sciatica, palsy and hysteria;
 HER: healing, arthritis and bedsores;
 R: now going on into the use of the oil especially in the treatment of old injuries and arthritis.

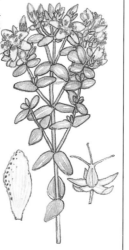

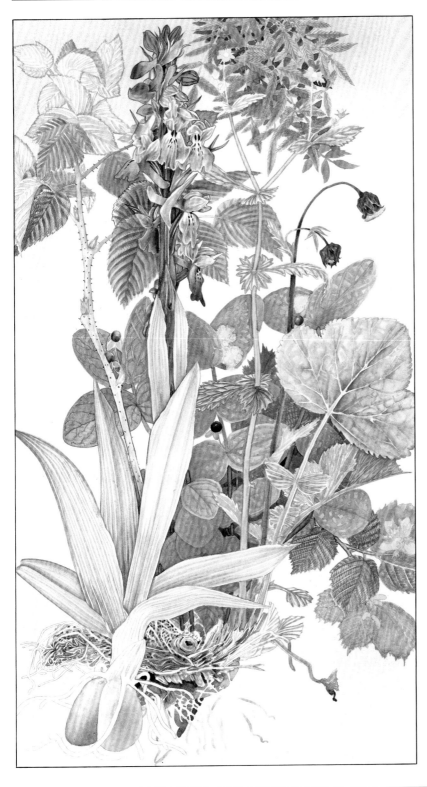

Limestone Woodland

1 St John's Wort, *Hypericum androsaemum*
2 Raspberry, *Rubus idaeus*
3 Early Purple Orchid, *Orchis mascula*
4 Wood Avens, *Geum urbanum*
5 Water Avens, *Geum rivale*
6 Ash, *Fraxinus excelsior*
7 Hazel, *Corylus avellana*

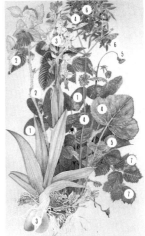

At the end of the thirteenth century, the Lord of the Isles, Angus Og, went to Ireland to find a bride. He returned not only with a wife but also with a physician, one Mac Betha. Descendants of the same, under the name of Beaton, continued to hold lands and practise medicine in western Scotland up until the seventeenth century. They had in their possession manuscripts which contained Gaelic translations of classical medical texts such as the Canon of Avicenna and the works of Hippocrates. These were copied again and again at great cost – sixty cows was recorded as the cost of copying one manuscript – but it was well worth it as they were the badge of medical office for the families of physicians. King Macbeth, in reality a commoner who usurped the throne and conferred with witches, was a member of this family. As research continues, we find that the Mac Beiths or Beatons of Scotland and the Myddfai of Wales have many links and several plant cures in common. The main link, however, is the tenuous line of temperate rainforest still found all along the Celtic coastline wherever it is wet enough. Rassal Ashwood, at the head of Loch Kishorn in Wester Ross, now a national nature reserve, is at the northerly limit of the chain which stretches up to the island of Skye, while a few Ash trees manage to grow on the Durness limestones in the far north of Sutherland.

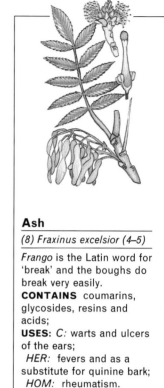

Ash

(8) Fraxinus excelsior (4–5)

Frango is the Latin word for 'break' and the boughs do break very easily.
CONTAINS coumarins, glycosides, resins and acids;
USES: *C:* warts and ulcers of the ears;
 HER: fevers and as a substitute for quinine bark;
 HOM: rheumatism.

LIMESTONE WOODLANDS

Ash-woods and Beech-woods, usually with an admixture of Oak, occur in their own right on limestones, especially in the south. They often have Hazel as an understorey, a tree whose dangling catkins produce more than their fair share of the annual pollen count.

The Celts associated Hazel trees with fire and fertility because that is how they cleared the forest: burning the trees and planting crops in the fertile ashes. When they moved on, Hazel sprang up to take their place;

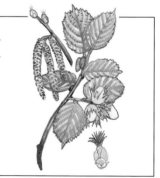

Hazel

(1) Corylus avellana (1–4)

Halloween was also known as Nutcrack Night, when hazels or cobs were used in all sorts of ceremonies of divination.
CONTAINS tannins and essential oil;
USES: *C/HER:* nuts sprinkled with black pepper have long been used as a treatment for autumnal coughs and colds, also used for menstrual problems.

so it came to be regarded as the tree of knowledge. In Ireland, a hazelnut carried in the pocket was said to ward off rheumatism and lumbago; the double or loady nut of Devon cured the toothache, while the same was used to drive away witches in Scotland.

Limestone woodlands, even those dominated by Beech, are often rich in Orchids which, although regarded as rarities, are members of one of the most widespread and successful plant families in the world. Beautiful and exotic they may be, but few have provoked much attention from the herbalist except for *Orchis mascula*, our commonest woodland Orchid, the Early Purple.

In the eighteenth and early nineteenth centuries, Salep or Saloop houses were commonplace and did a roaring trade in a 'mild and wholesome nutriment, superior to rice' made from the root of Orchids imported from Turkey. Who first cashed in on the fact that one of our own Orchids could do the job as well we shall never know. We can also only guess at what went on behind the façades of the less salubrious Saloop houses, for since the time of Dioscorides the plant had been held in high esteem as a nourisher of lust. The testicle-like structure at the base of each erect purple shoot, one remaining full ready for use the following year, the other emptying to serve the desires of the present, was both the root of the Orchid and the root of its specific Latin name, and in turn the root of all evil. What more could any man or woman want, as Robert Turner in 1664 commented in *The British Physician* that 'enough Orchids grew around Cobham Park in Kent to pleasure all the seamen's wives of Rochester!'? In the so-called Unicorn tapestries woven around 1514, *Orchis mascula* stands rampant purple against the white of the flank of that most fabled beast whose single horn was also reputedly an aphrodisiac. However, for centuries before this the women of Thessalonika had used the contents of the full sac to turn their menfolk on and the empty one to cool them down. By the seventeenth century the Diasatyrion, the official aphrodisiac of the London College of Surgeons, was more single of purpose yet of much more complex composition, as Geoffrey Grigson records in a gentlemanly way in his *Englishman's Flora*.

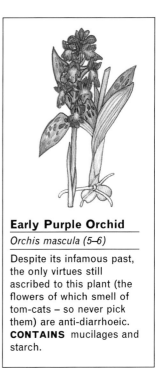

Early Purple Orchid

Orchis mascula (5–6)

Despite its infamous past, the only virtues still ascribed to this plant (the flowers of which smell of tom-cats – so never pick them) are anti-diarrhoeic. **CONTAINS** mucilages and starch.

This was made of Orchid tubers, dates, bitter almonds, Indian nuts, pine nuts, pistachio nuts, candied ginger, candied eryngo root, clover, galingale, peppers, ambergris, musk, penids [barley sugar], cinnamon, saffron, Malaga wine, nutmeg, mace, grains of Paradise, ash-keys, the 'belly and loins of scinks', borax, benzoin, wood of aloes, cardamoms, nettle seed, and avens root.

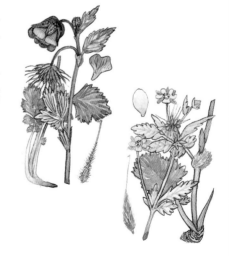

Wild Strawberry
(7) Fragaria vesca (4–5)

The woodland weed that was turned into the Strawberry of commerce. The little 'pips' on the outside of the fruit are in fact tiny nutlets and are a high-class dietery fibre. The leaves make a good black tea.
CONTAINS vitamin C, minerals, mucilages and essential oils;
USES: *C:* cure-all and tonic;
 HER: jaundice, diarrhoea, burns and depression.

Like so many aphrodisiacs of old, no modern proof of its efficacy has been forthcoming. Perhaps in these days of a good year-round staple diet, adulterated for those who need it with sex shops and steamy videos, there is no need to be reminded of the call of spring. Soft porn conservation in action for Early Purples are still common in the right places, though now much rarer than they were in Turner's time or even at the turn of this century.

The same is true of the next component of this electuary of our native woodlands, the root of the Wood Avens – an electuary is a medicine to be savoured with honey and other sweet things. Like the Strawberry and Bramble which still abound in our woods, the Avens are members of the Rose Flower Family. There are two types of Avens, Wood and Water. Herb Bennet is another common name given to the former and it is found in pictures and carvings decorating churches from the end of the thirteenth century, suggesting it was thought of as a blessed or sacred herb. It can be easily grown in the garden from its hooked seeds which stick to your socks. Its roots collected – but please only from the garden – pulled just as the plant comes into flower, have a pleasant clove-like scent and should be used as an organic clothes freshener and moth-protector. If you do attempt this experiment

Water Avens
Geum rivale (5–9)

Wood Avens
Geum urbanum (6–8)

Geum is Latin for 'give taste' and *urbanum* for 'city life', so plant it in your wildflower garden and do just that, add the 'taste' of our native woods to your urban existence.
CONTAINS glycosides which turn into an essential oil, tannins and bitters;
USES: *C:* cure-all;
 HER: tonic, and to aid digestion.

you will, I am sure, say 'A lot of labour for a little flavour.' In these days of instant spray-can everything I would have to agree, but in the old days when natural spices and perfumes had to be imported from abroad and were very expensive, this clove-scented reward was well worth all the effort.

Another now common member of the same family is the Raspberry which appears to thrive on disturbance, rapidly moving in to heal burned areas of woodland. In 1548 William Turner, sometimes called the father of British botany, recorded that it grew wild in a number of places on the Continent, adding 'They growe also in certaine gardens of England.' Despite this they are conspicuous by their absence from the plant lists of many medieval gardens. Fortunately they are today common both in the wild and in cultivation, for their leaves have now been found to yield a calming substance and are widely prescribed to ease monthly menstrual pains and those of childbirth. Perhaps cravings for out-of-season Strawberries and other fruits of the same family during pregnancy makes both home-confinement and homeopathic sense.

WET ALDER WOODS

Alder wood on constantly wet mineral soil, found throughout most of the British Isles, is the closest most of us will come to experiencing our natural forest. Whatever happens to a landscape, excess water must drain away somewhere and in the absence of concrete and culverts even the smallest streamside provides a wet-foot home for Alder.

Raspberry

(3) Rubus idaeus (5–7)

CONTAINS acids, vitamin C; the seeds contain 24 per cent fatty oils, and pigments;
USES: ornamental, cuisine;
 C: eyes, teeth, boiled leaves helped women in labour, and as an autumn tonic;
 HER: flavouring for nasty medicines, wound healing, diarrhoea.
 R: has shown that preparations of the leaves do aid relaxation in childbirth. The active chemical may be fragarine which acts on the muscles of the pelvis.

Alder

Alnus glutinosa (2–3)

Al is an ancient word for 'water'; *Alnus* the Latin word for the 'tree of wet places'.
CONTAINS tannins, resins and acids;
USES: *C:* sore feet, burns and inflammation, also against fleas;
 HER: the bark provides a gargle for treating pharyngitis and other sore throats.

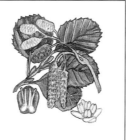

Pliny was the first to report that the wood stayed sound when immersed in water and builders and craftsmen put the written word into action. The Rialto bridge in Venice is supported on Alder piles, and drinking water has been piped into many great cities through hollow Alder trunks: urbanisation saw the machines usually used in the making of cannons modified to put a clean bore through Alder trunks which are very amenable to such treatment. Alder charcoal had already found favour as the best for making gunpowder; while the wood is such a good insulator that Alder clogs and sabots keep your feet warm and cosy.

Despite the fact that the roots of Alder are home to countless nitrogen-fixing bacteria, which live in large woody nodules looking not unlike clove balls, the habitat does not appear to suffer from too much nitrogen. Perhaps this is due to the running water which constantly flushes nitrogenous compounds away, for the gallery wood-lands are part of nature's own landscape-cleansing system. There are, however, a number of exceptions to this and certain plants brimful of 'healing poisons' do occur, although they are found away from the main areas of flowing water where nitrogen can collect.

Hemlock, with its purple-spotted stems warning of danger within, contains the poison once used to kill Socrates and one which has killed many since, thanks both to malice aforethought and to the temptation to make peashooters and whistles from the hollow stalks of the plant. Country lore records that animals, especially asses, which appeared to have died after eating Hemlock have during flaying, to the consternation both of them and their masters, awoken from the dead. An explanation may be found in Myddfai prescription 719 which records the fact that long before the days of Lister and modern anaesthetics Hemlock was used as part of a general anaesthetic.

The following is a potion which will induce sleep, whilst any diseased part is being opened.

Drink the juice of orpine, eringo, poppy, mandrake, ground ivy, hemlock, and lettuce, of each equal parts. Let clean earth be mixed with them, and a potion prepared, then without doubt the patient will sleep. When you are prepared to operate upon the patient, direct that he should avoid sleep as long as he can, and then let some of the potion be poured into his nostrils, and he will sleep without fail.

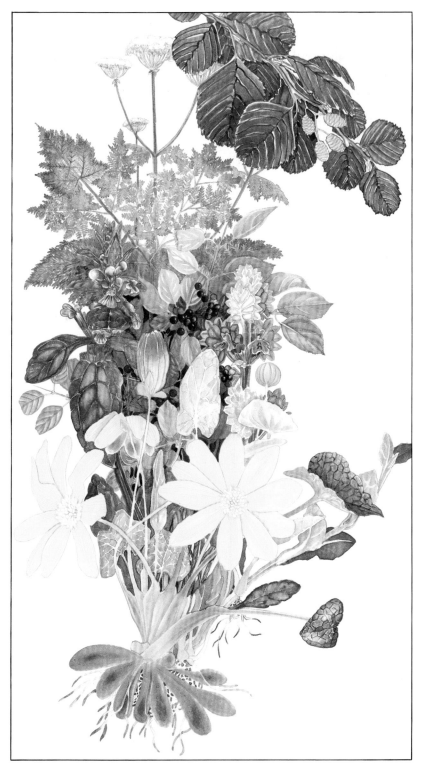

Wet Alder Woodland

1 Lesser Celandine, *Ranunculus ficaria*
2 Bugle, *Ajuga reptans*
3 Hemlock, *Conium maculatum*
4 Ground Ivy, *Glechoma hederacea*
5 Alder, *Alnus glutinosa*
6 Purging Buckthorn, *Rhamnus catharticus*

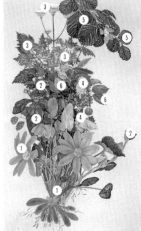

When you would that he should awake, take an onion, compounded with vinegar, and pour some into his mouth, and he will awake. Take care that you keep him quiet, and warned of the operation, lest he should be disturbed.

Hemlock Water Dropwort which grows closer to the flowlines is just as bad, or perhaps worse, for when brought into a closed room the 'smell' can cause giddiness and nausea.

Hemlock, *Conium maculatum*, is said to get its name from the Greek word *konos* meaning 'a spinning top' because, like the Water Dropwort, the first signs of poisoning are giddiness. Socrates, under sentence of death, evidently took his own life, as did many other ancients weary of the philosophy of existence. They garlanded themselves, giving farewells to invited guests, before they spun off their mortal coils by drinking euthanasic draughts of Hemlock. Conine, the active poison, was first isolated from the plant as early as 1831 and was the first plant alkaloid to be made in synthetic form twenty-five years later. It is still used in its pure form and in correct minute doses to soothe the pain of cancer.

While we are trumpeting success we must not overlook the beautiful and still common Bugle with its deep-blue flowers set against a spike

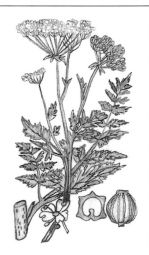

Hemlock

(6) (poison ×××××)
Conium maculatum (6–7)

The name comes from *hem*, the Old English word for 'border', and *laec* for 'plant'; a common plant of the damp borders of woods and fields. A plant to be avoided at all costs, it is a five-star poison. Let the purple blotches on the stem be a warning.
CONTAINS 5 alkaloids including conine, essential oils and coumarins;
USES: *C/HER:* poison, and as an antidote to other poisons;
  HOM: tincture, against hardening of the arteries and prostate problems;
  R: pure conine is used to soothe extreme pain.

Bugle

(8) (Poison ×) Ajuga reptans (4–6)

A in Greek means 'not'; *zeugon* means 'yoke'. Not a yoke around the neck of the people but a very useful herb.
CONTAINS tannins and a mild narcotic;
USES: *C:* a panacea for the digestive system, wounds, coughs, tuberculosis, spitting of blood, calming the heart;
  HER: gargles and as a wash for cleansing the skin;
  HOM: throat infections and rheumatism;
  R: insecticide.

of purple-black leaves: another of those common herbs which seems to have been used to cure all common ailments. Research at the Botanic Gardens of Kew has shown it to contain a novel insecticide which appears to work by sterilising the insects.

What other treasures await discovery in those plants which still make a trip down into the woods such a pleasant experience?

CHAPTER THREE

Coming down the mountain
❧

*M*ountaineering is a moderately modern innovation, indulged in by those with time on their hands and adventure in their hearts. There is, however, no doubt that across the centuries some members of every local community have been drawn to the top of their local high spots in search of food, a place of advantage or retreat, or just to see what was on the other side. These adventurous members of the local society were the first to discover that, as they ascended, the character of the vegetation gradually changed, trees became shorter and new sorts of plants replaced those which grew lower down. Upland and mountain forest, shrubs, and dwarf shrubs, grasslands and alpine rockeries were all set about with wet areas called swales where the rainwater is held back before tumbling its way down towards the sea.

So it was that the peculiar mountain plants, able to stand up to the rigours of long high-altitude winters and to pack their whole life-cycle into a short period of summer growth, came into the hands of herbal healers.

This appears to have happened only in the late 1600s after naturalist John Ray had written his massive tomes in celebration of God's Creation. He sang the praises of high mountains and the deep oceans, telling the world that they were not places of evil to be feared; that everything animal, vegetable and mineral, yea, all things were bright and beautiful if only we could see them in the understanding light of Creation.

At that time the mainstream medical tradition of Britain was steeped in the classical sources of literature. To try anything 'new' which did not have the authority of Dioscorides, Galen or Avicenna would have been looked on as foolhardy in the extreme. If plants could not be

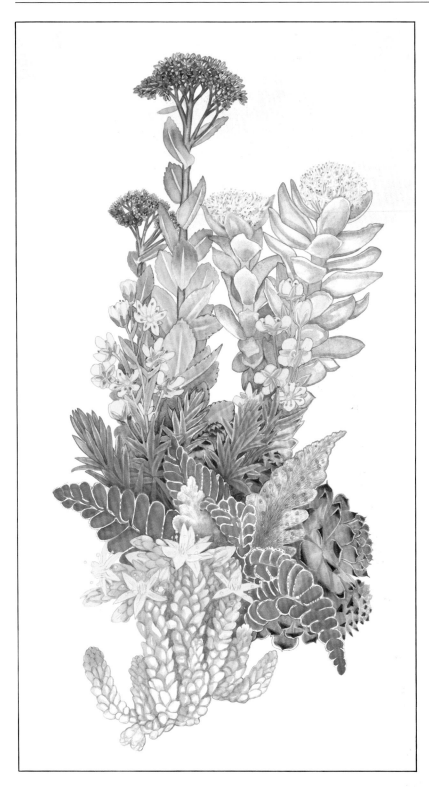

Mountain Rock Gardens, Walls and Roofs

1 Biting Stonecrop, *Sedum acre*
2 Rusty-back Fern, *Ceterach officinarum*
3 Yellow Mountain Saxifrage, *Saxifraga aizoides*
4 Orpine, *Sedum telephium*
5 Rose-root, *Rhodiola rosea*
6 Houseleek, *Sempervivum tectorum*

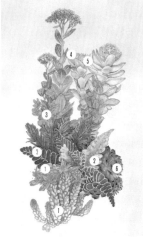

found in Britain which fitted the descriptions of these authors, then they had to be imported at great cost; or better still brought in as seeds to be grown here in so-called 'physic' gardens, that is if they could survive the climate. In the same way, if a local herbalist or wise woman used a plant that did not match up to one of the classics then it also would be shunned by the new professionals. In many cases this was done with good reason, for mistakes could be made and patients could die, but for others it was the stupidity of professional jealousy. 'People healing themselves? Preposterous! If that sort of thing is allowed to go on we shall all lose our status and be bankrupt.'

For these and many other reasons, few of our true mountain plants have common names of ancient origin, and even fewer found a place in the herbals. However, from John Ray's time onwards they do slowly creep into the literature of healing.

ROCK GARDENS

A very good way to bring the essence of the mountains into even the most urban of life-styles is to give part of your garden over to an alpine rockery, where a full range of plants which are naturally found from our mountain tops down to the montane meadows and forests can be grown with ease. Add a comfortable seat, preferably downwind, and there you have it, a year-round breath of 'mountain' air. One of my favourite places to sit and do a bit of rejuvenation is in the wonderful rockery in Edinburgh's Botanic Garden.

Please never be tempted to collect plants from the wild. They are rare and are getting rarer; they don't transplant well and the ones you can buy in a good garden centre have been selected and proven to do well in the down-town environment.

A good selection should include, from the higher reaches, the Least Willow, a good cover crop with wonderful splashes of colour when the vinous-red catkins burst open to reveal the white lint of their seeds. Its larger cousin, the aptly named Tea-leaved Willow, will do the same, thriving well at the water's edge. Mountain Avens really does deserve a better common name but no one seems to have bothered. Wait until yours has its silver-white fruits and have a local christening ceremony all of your own. The same with Viviparous Bistort; its name tells the botanist that it is programmed to be viviparous, which means that its flowers can bypass the luxuries of sexual reproduction and produce baby plantlets direct, so shortening the life-cycle, beating those early autumn frosts. Going by the other name of its lowland counterpart, Alpine Ledges, would surely be more fitting.

Shrubby Cinquefoil was first collected in County Durham and sent to John Ray who lived in Suffolk. Rare in the wild in Britain, it is so easy to grow that it has become a firm favourite with landscape architects, providing an abundantly flowering hedgerow and also shrubby genes for use by those plant-breeders who try to grow tall bush Strawberries, for both are members of the same plant family.

Meadow Cranesbill is still a common plant of our upland areas and, being found at lower altitudes, has a number of common names and uses in herbal medicine, healing both internal and external wounds. The same is true of the Bird Cherry which is used to this day by homeopaths as a sedative for headaches and for heart and intestinal troubles.

THE STONE-BREAKERS OF THE MOUNTAIN TOPS

These are plants such as the Saxifrages which appear to have earth-shattering powers, for that is what their name signifies, 'rock-breakers'. The fact that they often grow on bare rock or on gravel beside the clearest of mountain streams perhaps sowed the seeds of their use in cleansing the urine and breaking kidney stones, curing the dreaded gravels.

Nicholas Culpeper advised 'Breakwind helps the cholick and the stone.' Another name for the Meadow Saxifrage is Breakstone, and in its double cultivated form it is the Pretty-Maids-All-in-a-Row of the nursery rhyme. To be contrary, some writers maintain that the cures came first and the names followed, despite the fact that the leaves of many are kidney-shaped.

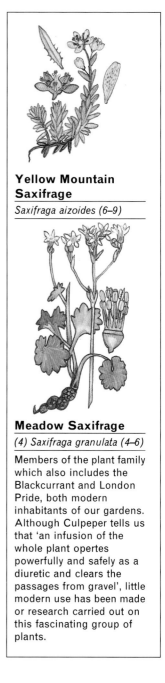

Yellow Mountain Saxifrage

Saxifraga aizoides (6–9)

Meadow Saxifrage

(4) Saxifraga granulata (4–6)

Members of the plant family which also includes the Blackcurrant and London Pride, both modern inhabitants of our gardens. Although Culpeper tells us that 'an infusion of the whole plant opertes powerfully and safely as a diuretic and clears the passages from gravel', little modern use has been made or research carried out on this fascinating group of plants.

THE BITTER BLUE GENTIANS OF UPLAND GRASSLAND

The most famous flowering plants which by their nature say 'mountains' have to be the oh-so-blue Gentians. Just as a walk in the mountains has always been regarded as an ideal tonic so too has the bitter element contained in Gentians, both blue and yellow. The members of the Gentian Family made themselves distasteful to the grazing animals which abounded on most mountains before people popped up on the scene by storing bitter-tasting chemicals in their leaves and other parts. These are so bitter that one of the chemicals, amaro gentine, when diluted in water one part to 50,000 still remains bitter to the taste. In the days before the extensive cultivation of Hops and when 'Queens and maids of honour drank foaming ale for their breakfasts bitter plants were in much request.' Sixteenth-century botanist John Gerard also mentions that a yellow species of Gentian was sent to him from 'Burgundie for the encrease of his garden'. The so-called bitters made from Gentians and other plants have been used as aperitifs since at least the time of Dioscorides, and are still used in cases of anorexia.

The fact that Gentians and many other mountain plants must store much sugar in their roots to tide them over the long alpine winters makes them ideal subjects for the production of alcohol for aperitifs. Gentianwasser, La Gentiane, Genziana, Goretschafka or

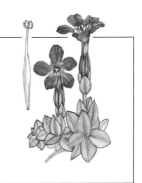

Spring Gentian

Gentiana verna (4–6)

Our only true Alpine Gentian, found in the wild in restricted areas of Britain although common on the Continent.
CONTAINS glycosides, other bitters and anthocyanins which make the flower blue;
USES: *C/HER:* tonic, aperitif, also against fevers and anaemia; Bach.

by any other of its many names would taste as bitter and make you hurry on to your starter to take away the taste. Modern research has shown that the bitter tonic stimulates the flow of the gastric juices which aid digestion.

A famous nineteenth-century finder and collector of our alpine plants was one John Binks, a miner of Teesdale in the County Palatine, who supplemented the income from his unhealthy occupation by

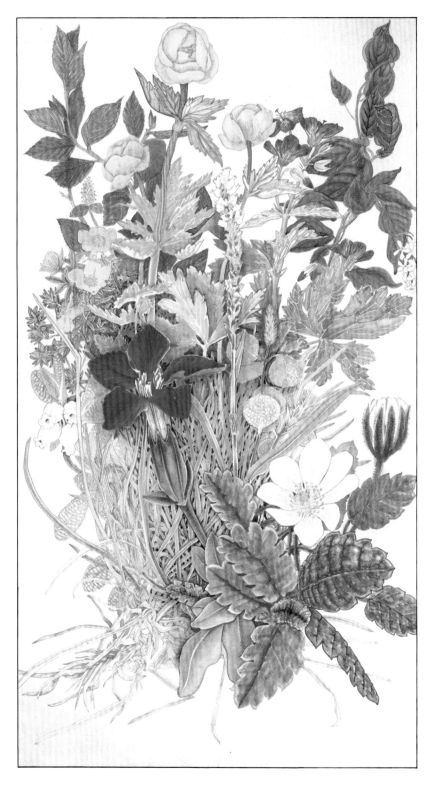

Limestone Grassland

1 Black Bearberry, *Arctous alpinus*
2 Shrubby Cinquefoil, *Potentilla fruticosa*
3 Tea-leaved Willow, *Salix phylicifolia*
4 Globe Flower, *Trollius europaeus*
5 Alpine Bistort, *Polygonum viviparum*
6 Wood Crane's-bill, *Geranium sylvaticum*
7 Bird Cherry, *Prunus padus*
8 Least Willow, *Salix herbacea*
9 Mountain Avens, *Dryas octopetala*
10 Spring Gentian, *Gentiana verna*
11 Blue Moor Grass, *Sesleria albicans*

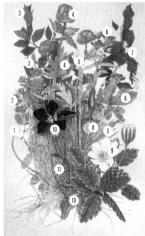

spending one day in every five at large upon the fells collecting plants. He passed the medicinal plants on to the local apothecary, the knowledge of his other finds on to the local clergyman and the local banker, James Backhouse senior, whom he had led on many a botanical ramble amongst the local Spring Gentians.

So famous is the Binks–Backhouse patch that the whole of Upper Teesdale is now a national nature reserve of international repute. Back in those days when wild flowers were still common, and even the gathering of the rarities was not a crime punishable by prosecution, the locals of Teesdale knew from experience that Gentians gathered early in the day kept their colour better than those taken in the afternoon or evening. The same is true of the bitters they contain.

BUTTERCUPS AND THEIR KIN

Another plant family which is common in the mountains, and should be handled with the care it deserves, is the *Ranunculaceae* which comes in many shapes and healing forms. Globe Flower (called Double Dumpling in Teesdale), Kingcup, Hellebore, Pasque Flower, Monkshood, Rue, Clematis, Baneberry and, of course, Buttercups must all be used fresh because their healing virtues soon fade away. Modern research has shown this to be true as the very active glycosides they contain rapidly break down to a number of simpler chemicals which, though still poisonous, are of no medical value.

This is a family not to be messed about with: handling even the commonest of Buttercups can irritate the skin and cause sores. Beggars

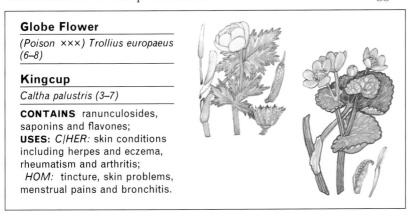

Globe Flower

(Poison ×××) Trollius europaeus (6–8)

Kingcup

Caltha palustris (3–7)

CONTAINS ranunculosides, saponins and flavones;
USES: *C/HER:* skin conditions including herpes and eczema, rheumatism and arthritis;
  HOM: tincture, skin problems, menstrual pains and bronchitis.

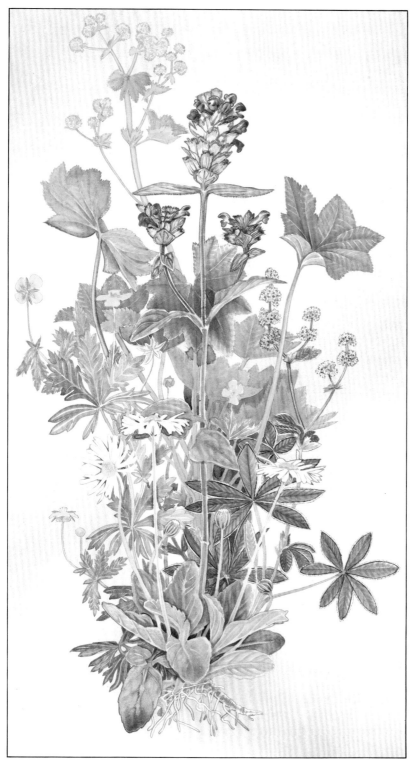

Upland Grassland

1 Tormentil, *Potentilla erecta*
2 Daisy, *Bellis perennis*
3 Lady's Mantle, *Alchemilla vulgaris*
4 Self-heal, *Prunella vulgaris*
5 Alpine Lady's Mantle, *Alchemilla alpina*

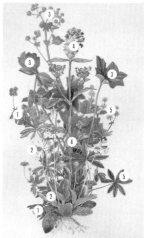

used to employ its poisons to give themselves rashes and blisters in order to gain pity and alms. Poisons made a virtue, at least to the giver. Today tinctures (dilute extracts made with alcohol) are carefully prescribed by qualified homeopaths to treat skin complaints including herpes.

Writing in *Flowering Plants, Grasses, Sedges and Ferns of Great Britain* in 1905, Anne Pratt says of 'Our pretty Globe Flower':

> Miller tells us that the Globe Flowers are gathered in Westmoreland, with great festivity, by youth of both sexes, in the beginning of June, and that it is usual to see them return from the woods of an evening laden with these blossoms, with which they make wreaths and garlands to adorn their houses. If this custom is still in existence, it will probably soon be extinct, for the old floral usages of our country, the flower-strewings, and the well-dressings, and the decking of houses and churches with wreaths, are almost over now, and even the garlands of May-days become fewer every year. The practice of dressing the 'shrine where we kneel in prayer' with funeral or wedding chaplets, though one of high antiquity, was early preached against by the Fathers of the Church, as a custom of heathen people; yet in country places it was long continued, and even a century ago these wreaths of flowers were very general. A writer in the *Gentleman's Magazine* of May, 1747, treating of flower chaplets placed in churches, says: 'About forty years ago these garlands grew much out of repute, and were thought by many to be a very unbecoming decoration for so sacred a place as the church; and at the repairing and beautifying of several churches where I have been concerned, I was obliged, by order of the ministers and churchwardens, to take the garlands down, and the inhabitants were strictly forbidden to hang up any more for the future.'

Fortunately, since those days of prudish austerity, the use of flowers in our churches has returned and the floral festivals and well-dressings in Derbyshire are again a glorious annual event. Fortunately, too, most of the plants, Globe Flowers included, are grown specially for the purpose, thus conserving the dwindling resources of our wild flower meadows upon which cattle used to graze with great contentment.

SELF-HEAL

Whether the early herbalists made a clear distinction between the mountain and lowland forms of our common plants is difficult to ascertain. It is, however, true to say that many cure-alls came from those commonest plants which can be found growing at every altitude.

Self-heal is one that fits the bill for it appears to climb every hill as long as the soil is not too acid. Like all common flowers it has many common names: Carpenter's Herb, Hookweed and Sicklewort, for it helps to cure wounds both large and small; Brunella in Germany where it was used to cure the Bräune or quinsy – an acute infection of the tonsils; while the French say 'No one wants a surgeon who keeps Prunelle'. Self-heal contains tannins which act as phenols: these are bacteriostats which means that they stop bacteria from multiplying. Self-heal also contains bitters and an essential oil and so provides an ideal ptisane, *Herba Prunellae*, which can soothe sore throats if used as a gargle although too much tannin can have the opposite effect.

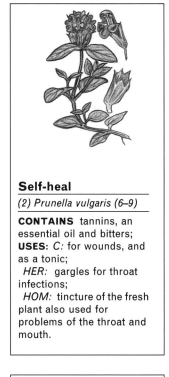

Self-heal

(2) Prunella vulgaris (6–9)

CONTAINS tannins, an essential oil and bitters;
USES: *C:* for wounds, and as a tonic;
 HER: gargles for throat infections;
 HOM: tincture of the fresh plant also used for problems of the throat and mouth.

TORMENTIL

Unlike Self-heal, Tormentil thrives on damp acidic mountain tops but is also rich in tannins; so much so that it was used in the Hebrides and Orkneys for tanning leather, one pound of it being equal in strength to seven pounds of ordinary (Oak bark) tan. The widespread digging up of the roots for this purpose so damaged the grazing on the Western Isles that the practice was prohibited. It is little wonder that the astringent properties of those same roots were highly prized to stem the flow of blood and also to stop up looseness of the bowels.

THE LADY'S MANTLES OR ALCHEMILLAS

Tormentil is a member of the Rose Flower Family as is the Lady's Mantle, which is found in all shapes and sizes from mountain slopes to the seaside. Lady's Mantle was Culpeper's favourite for healing wounds and staunching the flow of blood; the hairy nature of some of the species aiding the process of scab formation. From the shape of the leaves it gets its, dare I say, common name and its wide use in

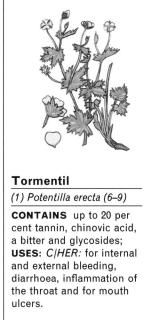

Tormentil

(1) Potentilla erecta (6–9)

CONTAINS up to 20 per cent tannin, chinovic acid, a bitter and glycosides;
USES: *C/HER:* for internal and external bleeding, diarrhoea, inflammation of the throat and for mouth ulcers.

beauty preparations and in tonics used during confinement and after childbirth to regulate the menstrual cycle. Pillows filled with the dried flowers were also used to induce sleep and so it came to be known as 'a woman's best friend'.

Although some say that the Alchemillas are avoided by cattle, Albrecht Haller, a Swiss scientist born in 1707, in his *Iter Helveticum* remarks that the extraordinary richness of the milk from cows in the Alps can be attributed to these animals having fed on this plant and on the Ribwort Plantain. It is more likely to

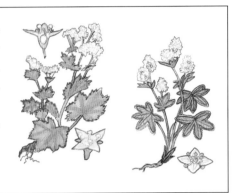

Lady's Mantle

Alchemilla vulgaris (6–9)

Alpine Lady's Mantle

Alchemilla alpina (6–8)

Taken internally and also used in baths and douches.
CONTAINS tannins and sugars; **USES:** *C/HER:* cure-all but especially for problems relating to the menstrual cycle and to childbirth.

be the varied diet supplied by the diversity of the alpine meadows which does the trick and recent research tends to bear this out. Cows, if proffered a natural meadow mix or a diet of perennial Rye-grass drenched with nitrogen, will choose the former. The name Alchemilla comes from the Arabic *alchemeych*, meaning alchemy, because early chemists believed that the shining drops of dew which collect on the leaves held part of the secret of the philosopher's stone which would turn base metals into noble metals – silver and gold. It was also considered to be an elixir of life, for Hoffman, a famous seventeenth-century botanist and physician, and others affirmed that it has the power of restoring beauty and freshness to the faded complexion when used in salves and creams.

The silver sheen and satin touch of the leaves of the Alpine Lady's Mantle remains even when stored for many years in a dried plant collection. This is a fact recorded by many botanists over the centuries, and so linked to its restorative properties.

FERNS

Before leaving the more open tops of the mountains, some of the groups of plants which do not bear flowers are worth a mention: first and foremost are the ferns.

High on the mountain rocks the Spleenworts can be found in some abundance. The Scaly Spleenwort or Rusty-back Fern was the most cherished by the old Arabian physicians. During periods of hot dry weather the fronds, which in warmer parts of even the British Isles grow with great luxuriance, shrivel and appear dead. However, as soon as humidity is restored to the air the whole plant revives in a miraculous way. The spleen was considered to be the seat of the affections, and so melancholia which could shrivel the constitution of even the strongest was traced back to that long thin organ appended to the liver. The passing resemblance and colour of the shrivelled fern fronds to the spleen perhaps gave the link, for it was claimed by the Ancient Greek physicians that 'Cretan swine when feeding on the plant lost that organ altogether, and it was believed that, when taken in excess, the same injury could be experienced by the human constitution.' Although Culpeper lists no fewer than thirty-nine cures for disorders of the spleen, this little fern gets only a brief mention: 'It is generally used against infirmitee of the spleen, helps the stranguary, and wastes the stone in the bladder, and is useful against the jaundice and hiccough.'

The action of the unwinding leaf would suggest its use against hernias and other twistings of the gut, while the changing colour of the spore mass links it to jaundice. Dioscorides was a great extoller of the Spleenwort's virtues which he counselled should be collected by night when, he believed, its virtues would be stronger and more active. Gerard gives short shrift to these old wives' tales:

> There be empiriks or blind practitioners of this age, who teach that infirmities of the liver also, may be effectually and in a very short time removed, insomuch that the sodden liver of a beast is restored to his former constitution again, that is made like unto raw liver, if it bee boyled again with this herbe.

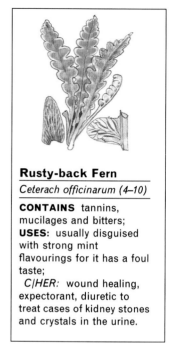

Rusty-back Fern

Ceterach officinarum (4–10)

CONTAINS tannins, mucilages and bitters;
USES: usually disguised with strong mint flavourings for it has a foul taste;
  C/HER: wound healing, expectorant, diuretic to treat cases of kidney stones and crystals in the urine.

This herb, or rather the fern, which up to the eighteenth century was listed in pharmacopoeias as a cure against jaundice was *Ceterach officinarum* – an official plant, as its name tells us. Extracts of its leaves were used in cases of jaundice until this century, despite the fact that the bad taste of the plant had to be disguised with aniseed, liquorice or some other strong-tasting extract. It was only in this century that an equally foul-tasting remedy replaced all others and that was the eating of raw liver; I can well remember my mother complaining about having had to do just that. The active element in liver, which unfortunately is destroyed by heat, is iron held in special organic form which is a key raw material for the making of haemoglobin. This haemoglobin is stored away in blood corpuscles – where else but in the spleen – ready to respond to all afflictions of the affections. All green plants store another metallic element, magnesium, in a somewhat similar and reactive organic form – the active element of chlorophyll. So perhaps those ferns which grow on the iron-enriched wet mountain soils deserve another less jaundiced look by the light of modern science.

CURES FOR MALARIA

Not all that long ago, malaria was widespread in Europe, including Britain. Known by many cursed names, the most appropriate of which was perhaps the shivering ague, the malaise was always linked to dank wet places where the cold dew gives off a silver sheen of hope as the sun rises afresh each morning. So, what better place to look for a cure than on the highest hills in your neighbourhood?

Having suffered from malaria while in Africa I can say with my hand on my heart that a patient would be willing to try anything to alleviate the symptoms and effect a cure.

'Take one Orb-web Spider and swallow it whole.' The theory was that the imprisoned bi-quadruped would then set about her work to build a web which, though made of pure protein, is weight-for-weight equal in strength to mild steel. So it will hold your shaking limbs together. However, whether an arachnophobe or arachnophile you might feel better both mentally and physically if you tried instead a decoction of the Common Daisy which can also be found growing on our mountains. Gerard's *Great Book* tells us 'made in water and drunk is good against agues, malaria and other fevers'.

Again and again, we find that it was the commonest plants which provided the curing recipes of the past. Homeopathy still employs an extract of the whole Daisy plant together with its saponins, essential oils, tannins and bitters, although in the past it was the flowerheads under the name *Flores Bellidis* which were mostly used.

HEATHERS AND HEATHS

One family which adores and adorns our mountains is that which includes the Heathers and Heaths. Although these beautiful and abundant plants have been adopted not only as a floral emblem of Scotland but also on badges of the Highland clans – Crossed-leaved Heath by Macdonalds, Heath by Macdonnells and Bell Heather by the Macalisters – their use in medicine has been somewhat limited; that is, unless their virtues have first been transformed and recycled by the honeybee.

We tend to forget that before the north-western world had access to sugar from the cane or beet, honey was the state-of-the-art food additive 'AP 40,000', for that is about the number of bees in a working colony. *Apis mellifera*, the honeybee, is without doubt the original homeopathic practitioner. Sipping the nectar and gathering the pollen from the diversity of local flowers, bees infuse the products of their

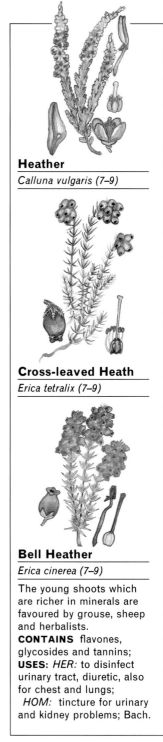

Heather
Calluna vulgaris (7–9)

Cross-leaved Heath
Erica tetralix (7–9)

Bell Heather
Erica cinerea (7–9)

The young shoots which are richer in minerals are favoured by grouse, sheep and herbalists.
CONTAINS flavones, glycosides and tannins;
USES: *HER:* to disinfect urinary tract, diuretic, also for chest and lungs;
HOM: tincture for urinary and kidney problems; Bach.

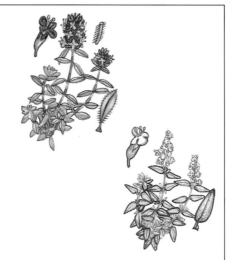

Wild Thyme

(2) Thymus drucei (5–8)

Garden Thyme
(2) Thymus vulgaris (5–10)

CONTAINS essential oil which includes thymol and cymol, tannins and antibiotics. The Thymes are treasure-chests of chemicals. Thymol is a powerful disinfectant and does not irritate the lining of the gut. Other constituents are calming and digestive. Used in medicines, salves, ointments, baths and bath oils, for anorexia, laryngitis and whooping cough.

labour with minute amounts of complex chemicals: homeopathic syrups full of natural energy and healing power, borrowed from the flowers.

The Wild Thyme on the mountain's knees
Unrolls its purple market to the bees.

So wrote Alfred Noyes, poet of the early twentieth century, for he knew that the apiarists of his times liked to put their skeps near those bald rocky spots edged with Thyme. This plant was thought by the ancients to harbour the souls of the dead and so its flowers were never brought into the house. This did not apply to the dried leaves, for they have been used since time immemorial to flavour foods. It seems logical to believe that a patient would have always been served, or at least tempted with, the best and most flavourful food available: instant energy and a strong taste together working the wonders of recovery. So, if Thyme used to flavour food encouraged healing, why not try the plant as a medicine all on its own; as an extract or in an ointment or cream? They did and it worked, soothing the sorest throat, thanks, we now know, to its rich content of thymol and *Ol serphylli*. To this day, chemists' shops still stock honey pastilles flavoured with all sorts of natural ingredients, including Thyme-honoured favourites. It is hard to sort out which came first, the curing of the folk or the folk tales that later became part and parcel of the prescription.

Cowberry, another member of the Heather Family, is a common plant of our uplands. It can be cultivated with ease and makes a good substitute for Box as edging plants or in parterres. It is still used, and is far superior to, the Redcurrant for making jellies to go with game and venison, and to make Cowberry tart, a local Derbyshire dish. Its near relative, the Bog Whortleberry, grows in similar places but is more plentiful in the mountains of Scotland. The leaves of this plant are said to produce a sensation of giddiness if eaten in large numbers.

Both Red and Black Bearberries have figured in the past in cures for various afflictions including the agues. The latter plants have nitrogen-fixing bacteria living in their roots and so enrich the plant and the habitat with nitrogenous fertiliser. They should therefore be richer in the nitrogen-containing compounds, arbutoside and methyl

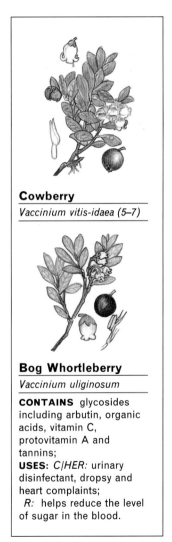

Cowberry
Vaccinium vitis-idaea (5–7)

Bog Whortleberry
Vaccinium uliginosum

CONTAINS glycosides including arbutin, organic acids, vitamin C, protovitamin A and tannins;
USES: *C/HER:* urinary disinfectant, dropsy and heart complaints;
 R: helps reduce the level of sugar in the blood.

arbutoside, than their red-berried cousin, the fruits of which go under the name of rapperdandies in Berwickshire. Ptisanes are produced by soaking the leaves in cold water but the product must not be used for fifteen days for fear of damaging the kidneys. It is of great interest that, under normal circumstances, the active compounds pass

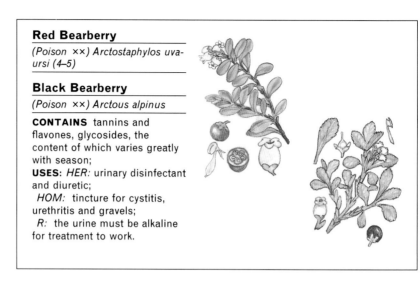

Red Bearberry

(Poison ××) Arctostaphylos uva-ursi (4–5)

Black Bearberry

(Poison ××) Arctous alpinus

CONTAINS tannins and flavones, glycosides, the content of which varies greatly with season;
USES: *HER:* urinary disinfectant and diuretic;
 HOM: tincture for cystitis, urethritis and gravels;
 R: the urine must be alkaline for treatment to work.

through the human body unchanged. However, if harmful bacteria are present in great enough numbers to make the urine alkaline, then the compounds are 'switched on' and become disinfectant; the bacteria are killed off and the patient starts on the road to recovery. Sodium bicarbonate is usually given with *Folia Uvae Ursi* to counteract the natural acidity of the urine and help make the Bearberry cure more effective.

Trial and painful error must have been the order of the early days but, once learned, the good news was passed down, first by word of mouth then in manuscripts and books.

Mistakes, however, are still made and yet another member of the Heather Flower Family, Bog Rosemary, warns the amateur not to meddle even in the mountains.

BOG ROSEMARY

Bog Rosemary, *Andromeda polifolia*, though rare and getting rarer in Britain, still grows in abundance in some spots in Scotland and other parts of Europe. Its leaves and its pretty pink flowers contain the deadly glycoside andromedotoxin, yet in Siberia the whole plant is used to make an intoxicating liquor. However, be warned, for death lurks even within the floral cup. The pollen of this plant is so charged with poison that the deadly nature of Andromeda honey has been

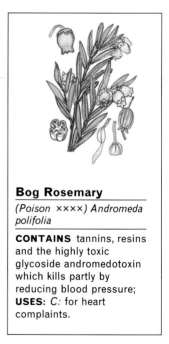

Bog Rosemary

(Poison ××××) Andromeda polifolia

CONTAINS tannins, resins and the highly toxic glycoside andromedotoxin which kills partly by reducing blood pressure;
USES: *C:* for heart complaints.

recognised since the time of the Greek philosopher, Xenophon.

The hard work of the honourable society of honeybees provides us not only with an energy-rich sweetener but also with several other complex products, containing a range of natural additives.

Propolis is a resin-like substance gleaned from trees and other plants and used by worker bees in the construction of honeycombs. Royal jelly is a special product compounded, with all the care it deserves, to be fed to those larvae which have been chosen to be the future royal line of ascent, and so lead a life of total commitment to the commonwealth of the hive. The queen not only lays all the eggs but also produces the royal 'wee' containing complex chemical messengers called pheromones which suffuse the hive with her royal presence; holding the structured society firmly together.

Bee pollen, so-called because it is a mixture of processed pollen and nectar moulded as a stiff paste complete with a soupçon of pheromone, is 25 per cent protein by weight. This protein contains all the amino acids necessary for healthy human development and growth: twenty-eight minerals, fourteen fatty acids and eleven carbohydrates. No wonder the queen bee deposits some of this precious substance at the bottom of each nurse cell, a starter kit for her offspring, a surefire launchpad for a b.. hard working life.

Honey and all the natural products which go with it are good for bees, and research proves time and again that they can do humans a power of good. Some bees can, however, do us a lot of harm: the sting of the honeybee can become an instant killer for those of us unlucky enough to be allergic. One strange fact is that the allergy commonly develops in the families, especially in the wives, of bee-keepers. The only explanation found to date is that the apiarist on returning home hangs up his overalls and other gear, well-spattered with bee-stings, in the warm kitchen. The active elements distilling off from the stings may sensitise the family, especially the wife, if she is the one who tends the wash tub or feeds the washing machine. All good bee-keepers should hang their gear in the garden shed and do their own washing. It is now possible for those who begin to develop the allergy to go to a hospital and have regular treatment with bee-sting venom, not too little not too much, and so build up immunity.

Of course, it is the plants that produce the pollen, nectar, resins

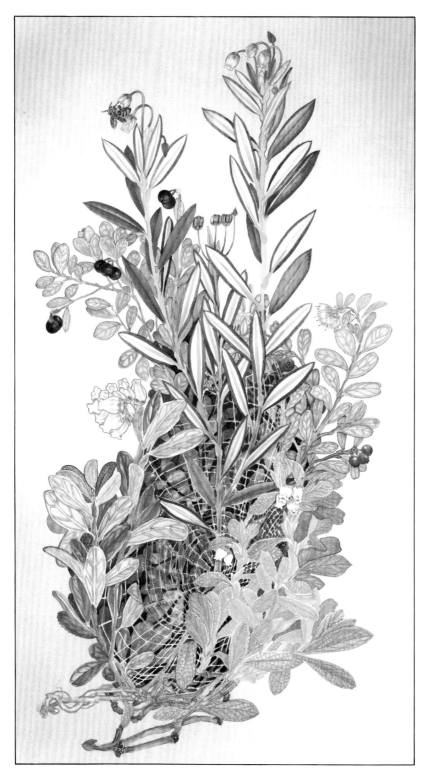

Acid Moorland and Bog

1 Red Bearberry, *Arctostaphylos uva-ursi*
2 Bog Whortleberry, *Vaccinium uliginosum*
3 Bog Rosemary, *Andromeda polifolia*
4 Cowberry, *Vaccinium vitis-idaea*
5 Black Bearberry, *Arctous alpinus*

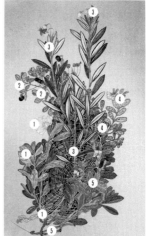

and all the other organic raw materials but, like the other animals on which so many people depend for their daily diet, the bees add more than a little something to their step in the food chain.

Climb every mountain, and wherever plants bloom, advertising their many wares to the insect world, there the bees will be found hard at work reprocessing the power of the flowers into all its energy-rich health-promoting forms. At night the bees return to the safety of their hives while the plants stick it out on moorland and mountainslope. As the nectar collects, it undergoes an amazing transformation: it begins to ferment and turn to alcohol. So it is that the bees on the early morning round may imbibe a little more than does them good and return tipsy to the hive.

HOUSELEEKS

Welcome-home-husband-though-never-so-drunk and Welcome-home-husband-however-drunk-you-be are the longest common names given to any British plant. The first is used for the native Biting Stonecrop, the latter for the introduced Houseleeks, both of which grow in abundance on the roofs and walls of old cottages.

The Houseleek certainly covered roofs in ancient Greece for Theophrastus himself noted, 'It grows especially on roof tiles where there is enough sandy earth.' The Romans called it *Diopetes*, a plant fallen from the God Jupiter to protect the house from lightning. Grown deliberately on thatch, it may well have helped to dowse the spread of fire or its many upright flower spikes could have acted as lightning-conductors. Geoffrey Grigson records the fact that even as late as 1952 (the year in which 4000 people died of smog in London over one weekend), a farmer's wife in Wiltshire still used the plant to make singren, a cooling ointment for burns, as had Dioscorides 2000 years before, 'great against ulcers, burning, scalding and inflammation'.

The derivation of those long and strange common English names is shrouded in chauvinistic prudery. In France, these plants with their upright flower stalks are called *Trique Madame*, referring to the cudgel or stick with which madam laid in wait behind the kitchen door. When anglicised, it became Prick Madame, a more welcoming reception however-late-you-be, and a reference to the use of extracts of these upright plants as aphrodisiacs.

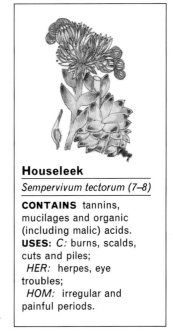

Houseleek
Sempervivum tectorum (7–8)

CONTAINS tannins, mucilages and organic (including malic) acids.
USES: *C:* burns, scalds, cuts and piles;
 HER: herpes, eye troubles;
 HOM: irregular and painful periods.

ROSE-ROOT AND ORPINE

Two other closely related plants which grace our high Scottish mountains are Rose-root and Orpine. Both, like the vast majority of the members of the Stonecrop Family to which they belong, have fleshy leaves bursting with sap and so are said to be gifted with aphrodisiacal properties, and both go under the common name of Midsummer Men.

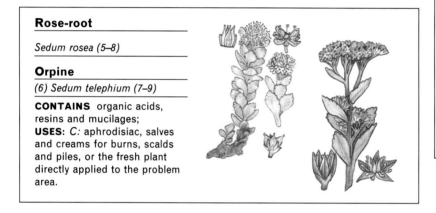

Biting Stonecrop

(2) (Poison ×) Sedum acre (6–7)

Can cause blisters and sores.
CONTAINS alkaloids, glycosides, tannins and organic acids;
USES: *C:* epilepsy, cancer, abortive, aphrodisiac;
HER: cure for piles;
HOM: tincture for piles and diverticulosis.

Rose-root

Sedum rosea (5–8)

Orpine

(6) Sedum telephium (7–9)

CONTAINS organic acids, resins and mucilages;
USES: *C:* aphrodisiac, salves and creams for burns, scalds and piles, or the fresh plant directly applied to the problem area.

In the seventeenth century the Orpine was grown, according to the antiquary John Aubrey, 'by Cooke mayds and Dayrymaids in pairs on the walls, one for such a man the other for such a mayd, his sweet heart', and accordingly, 'as the Orpin did incline to, or recline from the other, there would be love or aversion; if either withered or died, death'.

It is little wonder that these magical properties of heat and lust were transformed into virtues and cures. It is said on good report that Napoleon became interested in Orpine before he died of cancer on his lonely island.

The word Orpine means pigment of gold, which just goes to show that common names cannot be relied upon because its erect spike bears mauve-blue flowers.

ALOE VERA

Without doubt, the most popular plant with fleshy leaves used today is *Aloe vera*, a member of the Lily Flower Family and a plant from hot semi-desert places. The gummy mucilage from the base of the leaves was used as a sunblock by the people of North Africa long before any holes were discovered in the ozone layer. Today it is used in healing salves, especially to cure and protect from sunburn.

Passing down the mountain in the wake of those tipsy bees returning to their lightning-proof homes we encounter several plants which provide similar challenges for the human race.

Aloes

Aloe ferox, Aloe vera

Used since earliest times in North African medicine.
CONTAINS anthracenosides, aloin, aloe-emedine, mucilages and tannins;
USES: *C:* against burns, on wounds, as a laxative, and to ward off the plague;
 HER: constipation, also as a slimming agent and for burns and sunburn;
 R: as a laxative it works on the large intestine, but it should not be taken during pregnancy or if suffering from piles. *Aloe vera* is now one of the most popular constituents of cleansing and healing creams and lotions.

JUNIPER, BIRCH AND BARLEY

These three unrelated plants all undergo a change of character when their organic products come under the influence of a microscopic fungus called Yeast.

Juniper, though one of our four native conifers, is one of the few members of that great group of cone-bearing trees which don't produce woody female cones but fleshy fruit-like arils. Once fertilised by the abundant pollen blowing from tiny male cones, each aril, which starts its life as a green structure insignificant amongst the spiky green foliage, begins a rapid change. As it ripens it turns dark purple-black washed over with a floury bloom, and it is in that bloom that the tiny fungus, or its spore, lies in wait. The sole object in life for the Yeast fungus is to grow and multiply. To do this it needs energy from the sugars produced by other plants which it annexes to its own ends, and this produces alcohol as a by-product.

Exactly when people first learned to help Yeast to achieve its reproductive aims while themselves reaping the dubious benefits of alcohol, fire-water or the water of life, we do not know.

Wine was used to heal wounds in the Bible story of the Good Samaritan. It contains living Yeast and other fungi, especially in its home-made form, and these are all present in the fermentation vat. Many fungi produce antibiotics, 'And [he] bound up his wounds, pouring in oil and wine', as the story says, millennia before Alexander Fleming discovered the virtues of penicillin. Sealed amphorae containing details of vineyards and vintages have been found in the tombs of the Pharaohs; while the great medical papyri of the Egyptians, written more than 5000 years ago, add the virtues of wine to many of their prescriptions. A little of what you fancy does, or should it be 'dose' you good.

Despite the fact that the consumption of alcohol is forbidden by the Koran, its use for medical purposes is allowed and it was the natural philosophers and alchemists of the Muslim countries who brought the art of distillation into the arena of scientific medicine.

Distillation was first used in an attempt to extract and concentrate the hidden healing properties of animals, vegetables and minerals. It was hoped that this would bring about the transmutation of the four elements, earth, fire, air and water, and so discover the elixir of life. One early and great success story was the production of fire-water which, for the first time, allowed the production of tinctures – alcoholic extracts of compounds – which would not dissolve in water alone.

Across the ages each culture has learned the secret which provided them with their local water of life – arrack, armagnac, brandy, grappa or schnapps, a list which would be incomplete without two British contenders, gin and whisky.

Gin gets its flavour from the resinous fruit-like arils of Juniper. Its taste became addictively linked with one of the great all-time cures for malaria, Quinine. Quinine is one of those bitter bitters and it comes from the bark of the Quinine Bark Tree, a native of the rainforests of tropical South America.

So it was that the gin and tonny or, more correctly, the Juniper and Quinine, set came into lasting existence. It was this combination of plants which opened up those areas of Africa known as White Man's Grave, sending the word sundowner to the walls of extinction

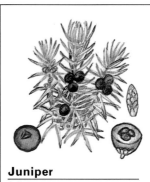

Juniper

(1) Juniperus communis (5–6)

CONTAINS essential oils which include alphapenene and camphene, organic acids, bitters and sugars; **USES:** *C/HER:* diuretic and digestive, urinary problems especially cystitis, rubs, salves and rubefacients (massage oils), also to combat loss of hair;
HOM: tincture for many diseases and conditions;
R: shows that this plant should not be used by people suffering from inflammation of the kidneys.

in an empire which spanned the world. Quinine is to this day a good malaria prophylactic, which means it can help prevent you from getting the disease and it can also help cure you once you've got it. It works by passing into the bloodstream and killing off the malarial parasite. Indeed, it is beginning to make a comeback as a malaria treatment because many of its synthetic counterparts are, in places, patently losing their grip on the local situation, the parasite having become immune to the synthetic drugs.

The Quinine Bark Tree is a member of the Bedstraw Flower Family, as is the Heath Bedstraw which grows in abundance on our mountainscapes, all of which are now affected by the debilitating ague of acidification.

Perhaps heath bedstraw was less common in the past before the days of coal burning and super acid rain, for I can find no mention of its use in herbal medicine. However, it is there to remind us that a weed is a weed only until its virtues are discovered; and remember that the virtues of Quinine were discovered by local healers of the Andes long before the Old laid claim to the New World.

Birch is a very British tree and one which thrives upon our acidic hills and mountain slopes. In its many shapes and forms it has long been associated with evil things: the Birch to scourge the wicked and the besom to carry the witch aloft. As if to prove it, Birch trees, when infected by certain bacteria, lose control of their growth and branch and branch again to produce large masses of twiglets which ride high on the branches deforming an otherwise beautiful tree. They grow under the name of Witches' Brooms.

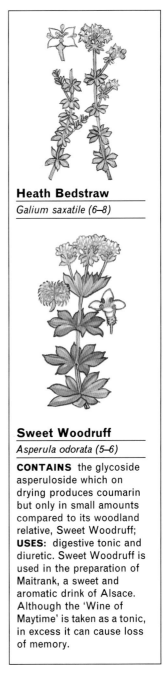

Heath Bedstraw
Galium saxatile (6–8)

Sweet Woodruff
Asperula odorata (5–6)

CONTAINS the glycoside asperuloside which on drying produces coumarin but only in small amounts compared to its woodland relative, Sweet Woodruff; **USES:** digestive tonic and diuretic. Sweet Woodruff is used in the preparation of Maitrank, a sweet and aromatic drink of Alsace. Although the 'Wine of Maytime' is taken as a tonic, in excess it can cause loss of memory.

Silver Birch
(2) Betula pendula (4–5)

CONTAINS soaps, flavonoids, volatile oil, glycoside and tannins;
USES: *C/HER:* diuretic, aids the heart, urinary disorders, skin creams and lotions;
HOM: rheumatism and dropsy.

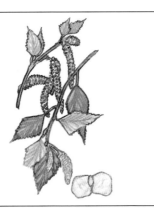

Mirror, mirror, on the wall,
Who is the fairest one of all?

Who knows, for in the language of the flowers the Birch is the symbol of gracefulness. So the trunks were tapped, and still are in certain parts of Scotland, in spring, and the sugar-rich sap collected for fermentation. Birch wine may also be made from the flowers and both were said to alleviate baldness, although there is no modern proof of this.

The third in our trio of the mountain tipples is Barley. A native of our islands, it finds a special place as a cereal crop which can be grown and ripened by our upland farmers. Barley is a part of another trio of natural products which includes branch- or rather burn-water and peat which provides the consumer with the myriad tastes of pure malt whisky. One dram is one-eighth of a fluid ounce and this imperial weight has been used to measure out correct dosages of each and every virtue with all the care and caution they deserve. One dram when taken as the water of life can surely do no harm. Yet there is always the danger of addiction gaining the upper hand and turning virtue into vice; the question of cure or kill will always hang over the demon alcohol.

Barley produces the malt from which the whisky is made. It also produces a whole range of soothing substances which, used in the form of barley sugar and barley water, have helped soothe throats and cool fevers across the centuries. Barley was an important ingredient of the Pharaohs' medicines 6000 years ago.

Study of a chlorophyll-deficient variety of Barley in 1935 resulted in the discovery of a new alkaloid called gramine. This led chemists to discover and make lignocaine, a very good local anaesthetic, and of great use to settle the heart back into rhythm after a heart attack.

Another cereal must be mentioned before we complete our catalogue of mountain cures: one without which a trip to the highlands of Scotland would not be the same. Oats are an important ingredient of both haggis and porridge, two staples in a healthy highland diet. Oatmeal, cooked as it should be to a porridgy consistency, bears out the 'doctrine of signatures' to perfection because, delicious as it is, the

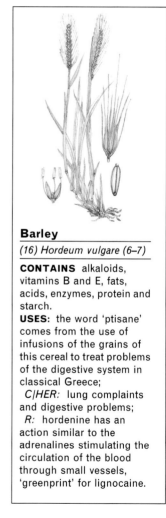

Barley
(16) Hordeum vulgare (6–7)

CONTAINS alkaloids, vitamins B and E, fats, acids, enzymes, protein and starch.
USES: the word 'ptisane' comes from the use of infusions of the grains of this cereal to treat problems of the digestive system in classical Greece;
  C/HER: lung complaints and digestive problems;
  R: hordenine has an action similar to the adrenalines stimulating the circulation of the blood through small vessels, 'greenprint' for lignocaine.

Oats

Avena sativa (7–8)

CONTAINS a vanilloside called aconine (which stimulates the nervous system and causes hyperactivity in horses), protein and fats. It is also a rich source of minerals especially calcium, cobalt, copper, iron, manganese and zinc, all elements essential to our life processes;
USES: good health, food, rich in body-building protein;
  HER: salve for skin diseases especially eczema; Bach;
  HOM: tincture, skin diseases, also liver, arthritis, rheumatism and paralysis.

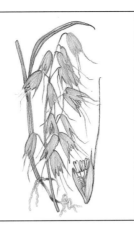

surface bears more than a passing resemblance to the disfiguring rash of eczema. Please don't stop eating porridge, it is great stuff, but if eczema afflicts you or a member of your family, try bathing them in oatmeal. It's an age-old remedy and it works for some as it certainly did for two of my children, one male and one female. There are a number of proprietary brands on the market.

There is one other plant which must be added to the list before we leave the mountains and especially those of Scotland.

SCOTS PINE

This is the tree that once formed the aromatic canopy of the Forest of Caledon, which itself once helped form and protect many of the soils of Scotland; reaching high up into the hills. Fortunately there are a few areas of this type of ancient forest still left in an almost intact state where, on a warm damp evening, it is possible to savour the true aroma of our highlands.

In Britain the Pine is a high-rise aromatherapeutic chemist's shop without equal. The whole tree produces essential oils, two of which were listed as official with their medicinal uses noted in the *British Pharmacopoeia. Ol terebinthinae* is extracted from the trunk and bark, phellandrine and pinene from the young twigs. *Ol pini sylvestris* comes from the buds, while the leaves contain carene, limonene and bornyl acetate. If that were not enough, in amongst all those exudations are the glycosides, pinicrine, piceine and coniferoside.

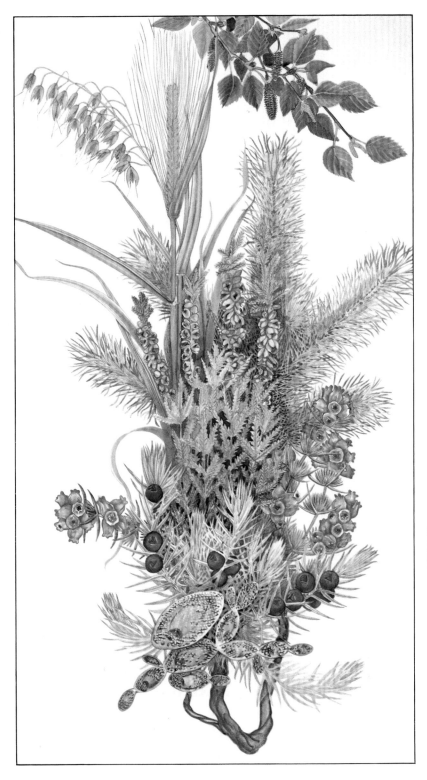

Waters of Life – flavour from the Highlands

1 Juniper, *Juniperus communis*
2 Scots Pine, *Pinus sylvestris*
3 Barley, *Hordeum vulgare*
4 Oats, *Avena sativa*
5 Heather, *Calluna vulgaris*
6 Silver Birch, *Betula pendula*
7 Bell Heather, *Erica cinerea*
8 Microscopic Yeast, *Saccharomyces cerevisiae*

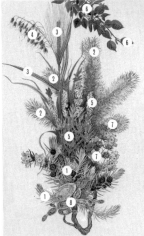

The uses of the aromatic virtues of our native Pine are in part thanks to the inspiration of two clerics who travelled in the New World colonies early in the eighteenth century. They could not have been more different in background: the one, Bishop Berkeley of the high church, philosopher and amateur doctor; the other, John Wesley, Methodist convert and revolutionary preacher to the people. They both returned from their travels singing the praises both of the health and the herbal knowledge of the 'Red' Indian people, and they both extolled the use of tar water, made from the resin which oozes from Pine trees. Berkeley made it popular with the upper classes, who used it for cold bathing, while Wesley took commonsense herbal healing to the masses. His pamphlet *Primitive Physic* sold well in the countryside, and especially in the growing towns and cities which were then gearing up for all that was unhealthy and bad in the Industrial Revolution.

Both, in their own way, took on the establishment of the day; the Bishop even suggested that clinical trials be conducted in one of the big hospitals. Two sets of patients suffering from a range of diseases were to be treated, one with mainstream medicines, the other with tar water. No one took up the challenge and tar water and *Primitive Physic* grew in popularity, much to the annoyance of the untrained druggists and trained apothecaries who were already fighting with each other for their slice of the lucrative trade.

The complex products of the Pine thus made their sticky mark on herbal practice, fanning the embers of an argument which still does nothing to help those patiently waiting to be cured by the best available method, mainstream or herbal. Today, both the argument and the aromatics are back on the operational table of modern medicine: used externally as liniments and baths, and in homeopathy in the treatment of chronic bronchitis, coughs, nephritis, pneumonia and sciatica.

The only word of modern warning is that patients suffering from inflammation of the kidneys should not use pine products. Then why, you may well ask, does homeopathy take the risk and use it for nephritis? Homeopathy employs minute doses of each chemical, so minute, some say, that they could never achieve any clinical effect. However, in the philosophy of Hahnemann, father of homeopathy, any patient is in a cycle of disease and healing through which the body must go. Tiny doses of a substance which may aggravate the symptoms speed the body into the cycle of recovery.

Please take a walk through what's left of the great forest of Caledon, along the shores of Loch Rannoch, and delight in the smell of those same chemicals. En route you might like to try Bishop Berkeley's Herbal Chewing Gum, oozing out of cracks there in the tree-trunks. Remember the warnings about kidney inflammation, don't swallow the resin, and dispose of it in an environmentally-conscious way.

A good treatment for those blocked sinuses is thanks to the wood-ant. If you are lucky enough to discover one of their volcano-like nests made from the aromaful pine needles, then gently lay your handkerchief on the surface of the nest. After a few seconds, shake well to get rid of any ants, and breathe in a tube-clearing draught. Have a care, for the formic acid produced by the ants can take your breath away. Also be careful where you put your feet or you may get a large dose of that same aromatherapeutic compound by injection.

CHAPTER FOUR

Water — the essence of healing

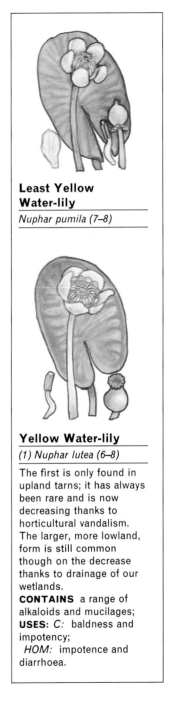

Least Yellow Water-lily
Nuphar pumila (7–8)

Yellow Water-lily
(1) Nuphar lutea (6–8)

The first is only found in upland tarns; it has always been rare and is now decreasing thanks to horticultural vandalism. The larger, more lowland, form is still common though on the decrease thanks to drainage of our wetlands.
CONTAINS a range of alkaloids and mucilages;
USES: *C:* baldness and impotency;
  HOM: impotence and diarrhoea.

*P*aludification is one of my favourite words; it means to make a landscape wet by impeding the flow of water as it moves down from the high spots to the sea. Springs, seepages, rills, rapids, waterfalls, tarns, lakes, rivers, meanders, ox-bows, swamps, marshes, fens, bogs and estuaries are all varieties of wetland which have fascinated me all my botanical life. Each has its own distinctive flora and each provides us with healing plants, and so they should, for rivers and their wetlands are the natural health systems of our countryside.

Like every other living thing, rivers pass from youth to maturity and beyond through five phases of existence: birth, initiation, marriage, rest from labour, and death. These are immortalised in the tradition of the Celtic people by the five petals of the Yellow Water-lily, a plant which in its two specific forms can be found from the highest mountain tarns down to the last meander of our greatest rivers, or could be before pollution took its toll.

THE SOURCE OF THE WATER

In ancient times the actual source of water itself was hotly debated because the link between rainfall and stream flow had not been made. Indeed, when the round Earth theory was first accepted, some argued that it was the pressure of oceanic water high on the curve of the planet which fed the mountain springs, the water being filtered free from salt as it was pressed through the rocks. It wasn't until Pythagorean logic linked the square of the catchment and the volume of precipitation to the flow of springs and rivers that an understanding of the working of the water cycle became possible.

Born in the mists, rain and melting snows, springs and seepages swell the run-off from the surface of the land. Falling fast over riffles and rapids, the water gathers momentum, tearing at and so eroding the landscape. It is here in the oxygen-rich headwaters that great fish such as salmon come to spawn the next generations of ocean-going young. Under natural conditions the erosion releases minerals from the rocks, helping to ensure that the sweet waters do not sour and become too acid.

It is all too easy to forget that we live on a planet, the surface of which is made largely of slightly acid aluminium silicate. Fortunately, under the natural conditions of acidity now prevailing on the land and in the sea, aluminium is held safe and does not dissolve in the water. However, wherever the natural balance is tipped too far, the aluminium becomes soluble with disastrous results, killing fish and other aquatic life.

THE LIVING RIVER

A river marries again and again, initiating erosion as it grows through the uncontained strength of youth towards the might of maturity.

Its main erosive work now complete, the river makes its way at a more leisurely pace across a flat plain which is in part of its own making. There the sands and silts, final products of the erosive process, are dumped, spawning paludification and so giving rise to ox-bows, marshes, swamps and fens in which the water flows so slowly that it becomes devoid of oxygen. This means organic matter does not rot away and peat begins to form, slowing the water still further until bogland begins to develop spreading acidity across the once fertile lowland scene. There is one great compensation: as the peatland grows and grows it locks up carbon into a long-term store, taking carbon dioxide from the Earth's atmospheric blanket.

It is in this penultimate stage of life that a river has much to teach us about the natural health of the landscape. A river and its wetland systems act as a gigantic kidney, cleansing the toxic by-products of erosion and of life, purifying the water again and again as it flows down to the sea. Given a chance, no matter how much organic matter, be it leaf-litter, animal slurry or human sewage, is voided into a river, the plants and animals of the flowing water will break it down and purify the water.

WETLANDS

Wetlands go one better for not only do they break down the organics and recycle the minerals they also strip pollutants and nutrients out of the water. One hectare of wetland can perform the function of £60,000 worth of a state-of-the-art waste disposal plant. Add to that the value of wetlands as long-term sinks for carbon dioxide, and nature conservation and environmental care become important facets of every economy.

Unfortunately it was not until many millions of hectares of watery wonderland had been destroyed by drainage, and many river systems had been so overloaded with pollutants that they could no longer perform their cleansing functions, that we began to learn the bitter lesson: the true value of letting nature take her own sweet course as part of the natural health system of which we should try to be a part.

RECYCLING

Each river ends its part in the cycle of life when its waters mix and mingle with the salt of the ebbing tide, as the submerged world of nymphs and naiads gives way to Neptune's realm. The river dies, to be born again once the cycle of living water distils pure clouds and rain to seed new life upon the dry earth, swelling the promise of each and every river.

Little wonder that amongst the plants which line the banks or grow within the areas of paludification there are many from which the ancients sought those with healing virtues.

Even today the fat rhizomes of the Yellow Water-lily still provide homeopaths with an extract used to treat impotence. Whether the alpine species, growing as it does nearer the source of the waters, is more potent has never been researched although we do know that an extract of the same organ of the White Water-lily, which is also called the Destroyer of All Pleasure, was once used as an anti-aphrodisiac.

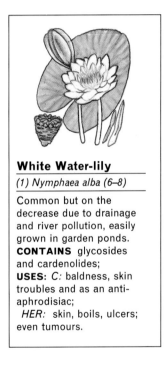

White Water-lily

(1) Nymphaea alba (6–8)

Common but on the decrease due to drainage and river pollution, easily grown in garden ponds. **CONTAINS** glycosides and cardenolides; **USES:** *C:* baldness, skin troubles and as an anti-aphrodisiac; *HER:* skin, boils, ulcers; even tumours.

CLOSE TO THE SOURCE

In upland tarns and lakes where the effects of the last Ice Age still scar the landscape, a number of other stalwart plants grow alongside the Least Yellow Water-lily. The Bogbean or Buckbean contains a number of bitter substances, and extracts of the plant have long been used to stimulate the appetite, cleanse the blood and cool fevers. It is one of the easiest plants to grow, even in a small garden pond. The beauty of its flowers when massed in the spring will do a corner of your garden, and you, a lot of good.

Ponds are a great way to add to the biodiversity of your own particular corner of Britain and also to bring the presence of these healing plants into your domain.

Water Lobelia is more difficult to grow but well worth the effort, for not only does it produce the most delicate of mauve flowers which shiver in the slightest breeze but also it reminds us of a very important healing plant of the past. *Lobelia inflata*, a more robust transatlantic cousin of our plant, was a regular import from America for many years as it was thought to contain a cure for syphilis, among many other things, and became an official plant used under the name of *Tinct Lobelae*. Our own plant, which is a rarity, was perhaps fortunately just too insignificant to draw the attention of our herbalists because it contains some chemicals which would make any patient vomit and perspire.

Our Bog Myrtle did not escape attention for it was a much more widespread and abundant plant in Britain before the mass drainage of our wetlands. It likes to grow with its roots amongst mosses, and especially in those places away from the main flow of water where acidity is just beginning to develop and where Bog Mosses such as *Sphagnum subsecundum* are just making their presence felt. Unfortunately

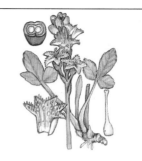

Bog Bean

(1) Menyanthes trifoliata (5–6)

A close relative of the Primrose Family.
CONTAINS bitters, mucilages, glycosides and minerals;
USES: *C:* many, including dropsy, jaundice, scabies and ague;
 HER/HOM: stimulates appetite in anorexics, a digestive and sedative.

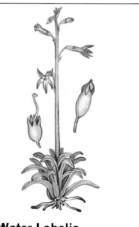

Water Lobelia

(Poison ××) Lobelia dortmanna (7–8)

CONTAINS alkaloids and mucilages;
USES: (American species)
 HER: syphilis;
 HOM: asthma.

Bog Myrtle

(1) (Poison ××××) Myrica gale (4–5)

Although in a separate family, it is one of the catkin-bearing clan which includes Birch, Alder and Hazel.
CONTAINS resins, tannins and alkaloids;
USES: *HER:* brewing and as an insect-repellent.

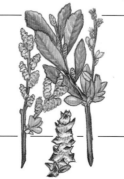

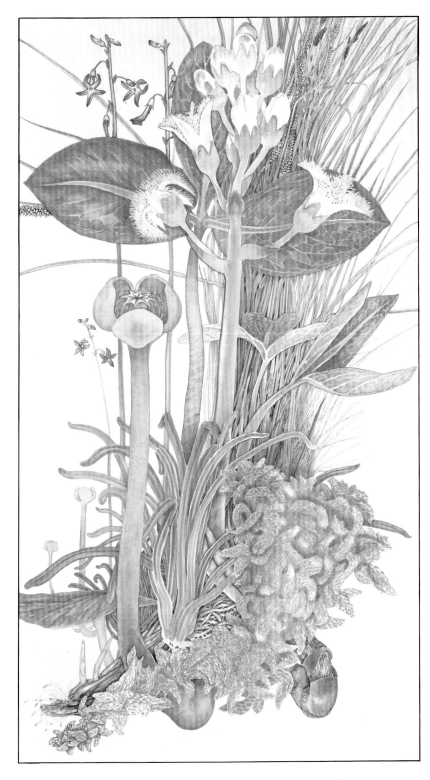

Upland Tarns and Lochans

1 Least Yellow Water-lily, *Nuphar pumila*
2 Water Lobelia, *Lobelia dortmanna*
3 Bottle Sedge, *Carex rostrata*
4 Bog Bean, *Menyanthes trifoliata*
5 Bog Moss, *Sphagnum subsecundum* Var. *auriculatum*

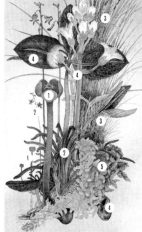

these are the very places which are first affected by drainage, and so today the Bog Myrtle is common only in our uplands and especially in the wetter west, although even there it is threatened by drainage. It is a small shrub oozing with resin which, on a warm evening, fills the air with a heady fragrance; hence one of its other names, Sweet Gale. Used with care in the brewing of beer, as it has some nasty side-effects, it was also employed in bedding to ward off fleas. Bog Myrtle is another of those plants which has root nodules complete with nitrogen-fixing bacteria and so is rich in alkaloids, a source of good or evil.

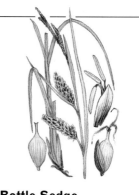

Bottle Sedge

Carex rostrata (6–7)

There are many sedges to choose from in Britain, they show just as much diversity as the grasses. Used only as hay and for litter, that is animal bedding, they have been neglected in agriculture and in medicine. We can only guess what virtues await discovery within this aptly-named plant and other members of its clan.

WHAT'S IN THE BOTTLE SEDGE?

Bottle Sedge, like all the Water Sedges, is not too difficult to grow around a garden pond and produces ideal launchpads for the dragon-flies and damselflies which will soon come to enjoy your own mini-nature reserve. The sedges, like the grasses, do not have showy coloured flowers and so are often thought to be less interesting and more difficult to identify. The grasses not only feed us in the form of cereals and dairy products, once they have been processed by cows and sheep, but they quickly cover exposed soils thus healing scars and preventing erosion. Although the sedges don't directly provide us with any food, they are of immense importance in the wetland and upland habitats where they often dominate the vegetation, protecting the soil and feeding the animals. As far as I can ascertain, only one of our own native sedges has been employed in herbal medicine and we shall find it at the end of our journey down the wetland way. So, to begin at the beginning.

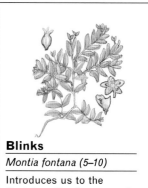

Blinks

Montia fontana (5–10)

Introduces us to the Portulaca Family, many of which are used as pot herbs. One reason for its strange common name may be that the tiny white flowers rarely open. **CONTAINS** mucilages, resins and minerals.

SPRINGS AND SPRING TONICS

Upland springs are often dominated by two curious little herbs called Blinks and Brooklime. I can find no account of the use of the first in medicine, and its common name appears to be much more of a mystery than its Latin binomial *Montia fontana*. Perhaps it comes from the fact that as the water wells up from the fountains in the mountains the multitude of leaves appear to blink, thousands of green eyes blinking away the tears of another day.

Brooklime, *Veronica beccabunga*, is a much commoner plant and does its best to bung up springs and becks alike. At one time it was used as commonly as Watercress for it contains in its many forms a goodly proportion of the minerals and vitamins listed on the daily cereal packet. It is used to this day as a springtime tonic and diuretic.

Brooklime

Veronica beccabunga (5–9)

CONTAINS bitters and glycosides;
USES: As salads;
 C: tonic, soothing coughs, diuretic (increases the output of urine), jaundice and skin complaints, anti-scurvy;
 HER/HOM: diuretic, liver and skin conditions.

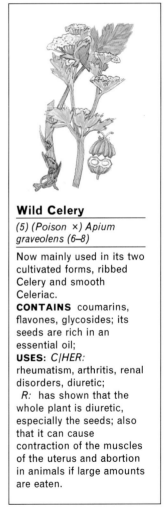

Brooklime introduces us to the whole complex of Speedwells, which are found from our mountain tops down to all but the best-kept lawns beside the sea. With a name like Speedwell, it just has to do you good and so it did, for in 1690 Johannes Francus, herbalist, produced the *Pulchresta, Herba Veronica*, a 300-page treatise extolling its many virtues in dealing with bronchitis, pruritis and infections of the skin. *Veronica* has both Latin *vern* and Greek *icon* roots and means 'true image'. Legend has it that the handkerchief of Saint Veronica was used to wipe the sweat from Christ's brow as he made his way to Calvary, so the piece of cloth and the flower bear the image of the face of Christ.

This parable was passed down by word of mouth to explain the miracle of healing lodged in this common flower. Country people knew the signs to look for and so avoided collecting other plants such as Hemlock Water Dropwort, a deadly poisonous herb which grows in similar places and is even more deadly than the bleeding gums, rotten teeth and stinking breath which characterise scurvy, the disease which Brooklime helped to cure.

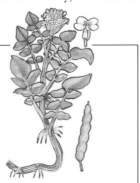

Watercress

(10) Nasturtium officinale (6–8)

From the Anglo-Saxon 'ea-cerse' – water cress, or 'wielle-cerse' – well cress.
CONTAINS bitters, vitamins C and F, iron and iodine;
USES: *C:* spring tonic, scurvy, coughs, bronchitis and skin diseases. Still one of the most popular year-round salads.

Wild Celery

(5) (Poison ×) Apium graveolens (6–8)

Now mainly used in its two cultivated forms, ribbed Celery and smooth Celeriac.
CONTAINS coumarins, flavones, glycosides; its seeds are rich in an essential oil;
USES: *C/HER:* rheumatism, arthritis, renal disorders, diuretic;
 R: has shown that the whole plant is diuretic, especially the seeds; also that it can cause contraction of the muscles of the uterus and abortion in animals if large amounts are eaten.

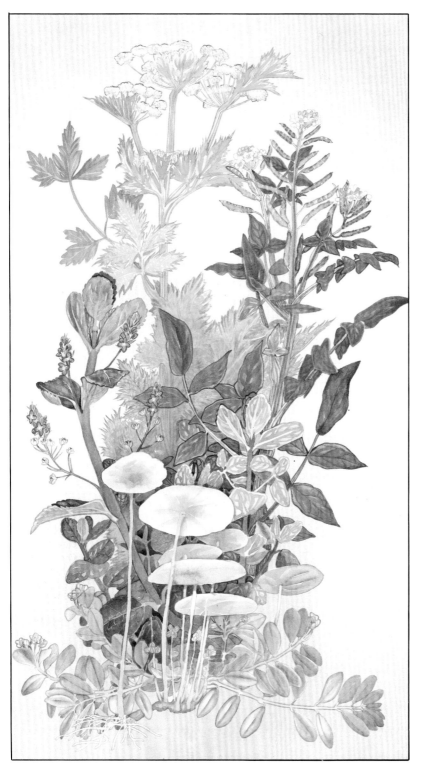

Springs and Springheads

1 Blinks, *Montia fontana*
2 Brooklime, *Veronica beccabunga*
3 Wild Celery, *Apium graveolens*
4 Watercress, *Nasturtium officinale*
5 Marsh Pennywort, *Hydrocotyle vulgaris*

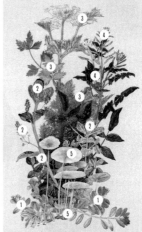

Scurvy had always been a curse of people, especially those who lived in a temperate climate where, at the end of a long winter, fresh greens full of vitamin C were always in short supply. Thus it was that in the thirteenth century Lemocton, now Lemmington, in Northumberland became an important place as valuable Brooklime grew there. Later, special water-gardens were set up to grow Watercresses. The first on official record was in 1808 on the Kentish side of the then expanding London, through whose streets the cry of 'Buy my fresh cresses' rang even in the depths of winter.

At the same time that Watercress gardens were springing up all around our expanding cities, great rivers such as the Thames had become open sewers. The pollution load was so great that the natural processes of microlife could no longer cleanse the water. So bad did it become that blankets soaked in phenol had to be hung at the windows of the Palace of Westminster to keep away the stench and protect the honourable members within from the disease without. Meanwhile, out in the countryside rivers still flowed pure and free and life went on as it had over the centuries, each local herbalist knowing the special spots to visit and each year reaping a sustainable harvest of health.

STREWING HERBS

Long before the days of wall-to-wall fitted carpets, the floors of castles, stately homes and cottages were covered with Strewing Rushes. These not only softened the tread on the stone flags but freshened the air with a variety of pleasant scents and as they composted they warmed the feet in winter. The poorer people used whatever came to hand and in those days the common rushes which now plague all badly-drained land were perhaps kept in check by this annual harvest. Even today there are in the Pennines, in places such as Warcop, annual church services which bless these humble plants before they are laid in the church. One plant which was always included in these rush mats and carpets was Meadowsweet, a plant which goes under a number of other common names: Courtship and Matrimony, Goat's Beard, Queen of the Meadow, and many more. As Gerard wrote, 'The leaves and flowers far excell all other strowing herbes, for to

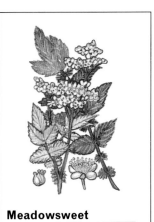

Meadowsweet

(3) Filipendula ulmaria (7–8)

CONTAINS the greenprint (a green blueprint) for aspirin, also contains tannins and coumarins;
USES: *C:* to flavour mead, wine, beer and soups; said to be good for the stomach; flour made from the root used in bread making; the root also provides a good black dye;
 HER: rheumatism, arthritis, water retention causing swelling of the limbs, and urinary infections.

decke up houses, for the smell thereof make the hart merrie, deligteth the senses, neither does it cause headach or loathsomness to meate, as some other sweete smelling herbes do.'

Just as later carpets were imported from the East to decorate and insulate our homes, so too was the Gladdon or Sweet Flag, a plant of India, where the rhizomes, which have a pungent sweet-smelling rind, were sold in the bazaars. The plant was known to Dioscorides and was introduced into Europe via Turkey in 1567. Soon after, Gerard grew it in London whence it escaped or was transplanted far and wide across the country. It is today a popular item at our garden centres in the water department. If you get the conditions right in your garden pond it will multiply and tend to take over. This is the time to try strewing it on your kitchen floor or, better still, candy the rind and keep it handy to soothe heartburn of the stomach, and so gladden your constitution.

FLAGS AND LOOSESTRIFES

Yellow Flag is another plant of the water which, if given a chance, will take over your pond and act as a year-by-year reminder of the problem of an exploding population. Do not confuse it with the Stinking Iris, whose flags, once crushed, smell somewhat of rotten meat, and whose flowers are grey-purple, rarely yellow. The Stinking Iris is also much less of a waterside plant but reposes in damp rushy patches, especially on mountains and near the coast. Used at least since Anglo-Saxon times as a good purge when steeped in ale, both were looked upon as apotropaic plants which, hung about the doors of churches and homes, were supposed to avert evil.

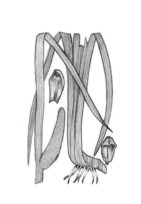

Sweet Flag

(3) (Poison ×) Acorus calamus (5–7)

One of the commonest medicines sold in the bazaars of India even today; it used to be imported into Britain to treat many disorders. Best known as a night nurse, a Vick-like chest-rub for children and for rheumatic joints.
CONTAINS aromatic bitters, antibiotics and tannin;
USES: *HER:* dyspepsia, anorexia, flatulence and indigestion.

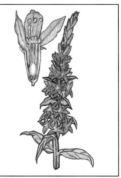

Purple Loosestrife

Lythrum salicaria (7–8)

Lythrum comes from the Greek word for blood.
CONTAINS tannins, pectins and an essential oil;
USES: roots for tanning leather, shoots give a black hair dye;
 C: eye-wash to preserve and strengthen sight, ointments for wounds and ulcers, to which fresh leaves were also applied;
 HER: anti-diarrhoea and dysentery, and in vaginal douches.

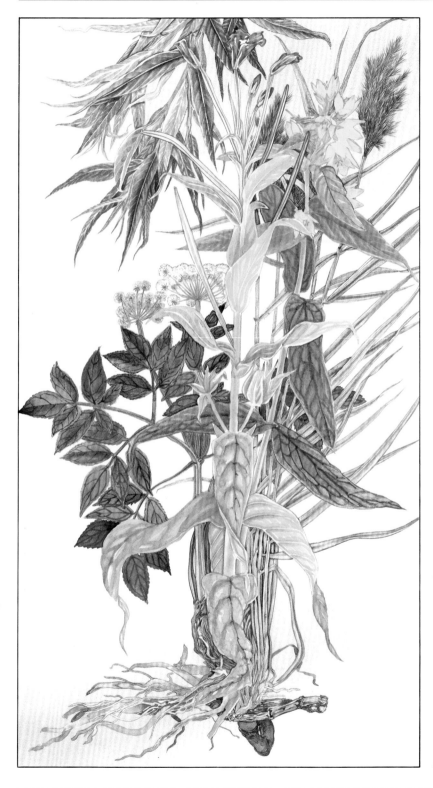

Rivers and Streamsides

1 Angelica, *Angelica sylvestris*
2 Cricket Bat Willow, *Salix alba*
   Var. *caerulea*
3 Great Hairy Willowherb,
   Epilobium hirsutum
4 Yellow Loosestrife, *Lysimachia
   vulgaris*
5 Common Reed, *Phragmites
   australis*

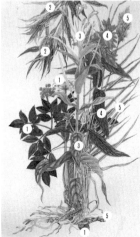

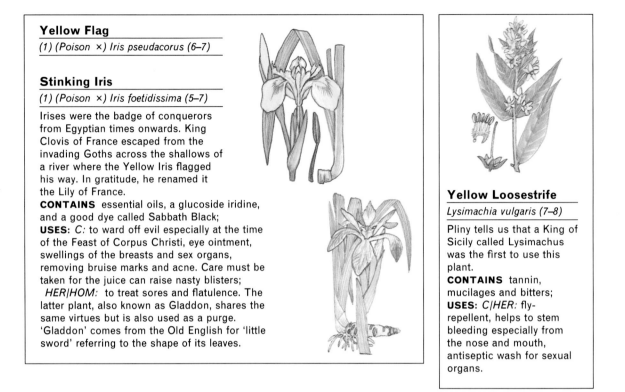

Yellow Flag
(1) (Poison ×) Iris pseudacorus (6–7)

Stinking Iris
(1) (Poison ×) Iris foetidissima (5–7)

Irises were the badge of conquerors from Egyptian times onwards. King Clovis of France escaped from the invading Goths across the shallows of a river where the Yellow Iris flagged his way. In gratitude, he renamed it the Lily of France.
CONTAINS essential oils, a glucoside iridine, and a good dye called Sabbath Black;
USES: *C:* to ward off evil especially at the time of the Feast of Corpus Christi, eye ointment, swellings of the breasts and sex organs, removing bruise marks and acne. Care must be taken for the juice can raise nasty blisters;
HER/HOM: to treat sores and flatulence. The latter plant, also known as Gladdon, shares the same virtues but is also used as a purge. 'Gladdon' comes from the Old English for 'little sword' referring to the shape of its leaves.

Yellow Loosestrife
Lysimachia vulgaris (7–8)

Pliny tells us that a King of Sicily called Lysimachus was the first to use this plant.
CONTAINS tannin, mucilages and bitters;
USES: *C/HER:* fly-repellent, helps to stem bleeding especially from the nose and mouth, antiseptic wash for sexual organs.

Two waterside plants which are again separated by flower colour yet linked by name are the Yellow and Purple Loosestrife. The latter is a member of the Loosestrife Flower Family; the former is a member of the Primrose Family. The name Loosestrife comes from the Greek *lusmachion* which means ending strife, and both plants were used to calm horses and oxen when yoked together. The fact that both were also burned to drive away flies and gnats suggests some insect-repellent properties. No wonder they helped the animals.

WILLOW CARRS

In the days when our water meadows, marshes and fens were part of every countryside economy they were cut each year to provide thatch, strewing herbs, animal bedding and a host of other useful things. If left uncut they soon became choked with ranker growth and eventually became wet woodland, as will your garden pond if left to nature's own devices. The stage of colonisation between water and woodland has its own special name, carr, and in its earlier stages is dominated by Willow bushes then, as time passes, by trees.

The Willows come in many species, shapes and forms and so have been used for several purposes including osiers for making baskets and great mats

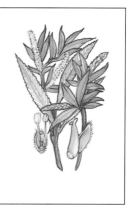

Cricket Bat Willow

(2) Salix alba var. *caerulea (4–5)*

The fact that the bark of Willows gave rapid relief to headaches and to fevers of all sorts has been known at least since the times of Ancient Greece.
CONTAINS glycosides, salicin, salicortine and tannins;
USES: *C/HER/HOM:* tonic, reducing fever, headaches and for rheumatism; Bach.
R: ongoing into treating ovarian congestion, and its calming effect on nervous excitement, especially of the digestive system.

used for strengthening the banks of rivers, dykes and ditches. Some of the latter which were laid down in Roman times are still doing their job today, while the former are now coming back into their own replacing the polythene bag in new-age sustainable shopping. Then, of course, there is the Cricket Bat Willow which adds that special summer Saturday sound which is almost as much a part of the English countryside as the wind in the Willows themselves. It is a wind which has blown everyone a lot of good because safe within the bark of the tree is a bitter substance, salicin, first used as a cheap substitute for Quinine by the Reverend Edward Stone in 1763. From then on it was used in cases of acute rheumatic fever. Only later was it proved that the human body converts the salicin to salicylic acid, the active ingredient of aspirin. This pain-reliever was first extracted from Meadowsweet and introduced in its synthesised form, acetyl salicylic acid, in 1899, since when it has been doing both our heads and, more recently it has been found, our hearts a lot of good.

The Willow-herbs, which have leaves like Willows, are members of yet another family to which they give their name. In the Second World War many Londoners came to know them as healing herbs because the Rosebay or Fireweed, introduced from America as a garden plant probably early in the seventeenth century, took over bomb sites and covered some of the scars of war. The Great Hairy Willow-herb, or Codlins-and-Cream, is a plant of the Willow carr. Its second name comes from the colour of its flowers, each one like a rosy codlin apple with a dob of cream on top, the flower and the white stigma attracting insects and people alike.

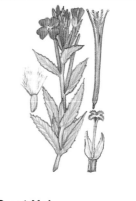

Great Hairy Willow-herb

Epilobium hirsutum (7–8)

A very common plant which could not have gone unnoticed for it grows about mill-streams, hence another of its names, Milner Flower.
CONTAINS tannins, pectins and mucilages;
USES: none, although Linnaeus suggested that the leaves of some species can be eaten as a salad and the young shoots served like Asparagus.

VILLAGE PONDS

Even the humble village pond used over the centuries to water horses and other animals provides a wealth of healing plants.

Bistort is called Easter Ledges in the Lake District, where a pudding is still made from its leaves and eaten at Eastertide or during Lent. Bistort, the plant of virtue, means 'to cause to retayne and conceyve', according to Gerard in 1526.

Growing alongside this may be found Persicaria or Adam's Plaster, a plant of lesser virtue for the twin black marks which bruise its leaves are said to have been made by the Virgin Mary who picked it, perhaps from below the cross, but finding it of no use cast it away. Perhaps she mistook it for its much larger brother, the Water Pepper, which can grow in similar places. Both are also known by the name of arsesmart, and certainly the latter 'if laid upon the tayle or other bare

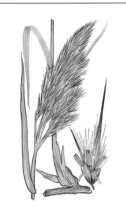

Common Reed

Phragmites australis (8–9)

As its common name implies, it is found the world over in damp places and along the sides of rivers. It is one of the great healers of our river banks and cleansers of their waters. Reed thatching has long protected people from the elements and reedbeds are now being built for the final treatment of sewage and other effluents.
CONTAINS silica, antibiotics and mucilages;
USES: *C:* to draw splinters and thorns, against scurf and loss of hair. The leaves were also used as a sharp blade to cut the umbilical cord and so start many human beings into a new cycle of life.

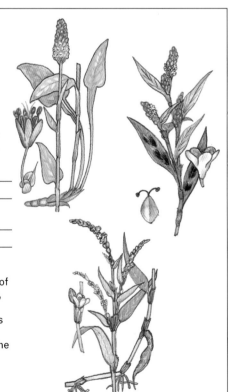

Bistort

Polygonum bistorta (6–8)

A member of the plant family which gave the world of medicine the virtues of Rhubarb.
CONTAINS tannins, mucilages and resins;
USES: *C:* to help painful periods, treat diarrhoea and also to aid conception and childbirth.

Persicaria

(1) Polygonum persicaria (6–10)

Water Pepper

Polygonum hydropiper (7–9)

CONTAIN essential oils, flavones and tannins;
USES: *C/HER:* used for a range of complaints from chronic eczema, through jaundice to arthritis and lung problems. The latter plant is thought to be the *Hydropeperi* of Dioscorides, which was one of the universal remedies of Classical times. Still used today as a flea-repellent.

skinne, it maketh it smart', warns Gerard. Yet it was laid green upon the bed to kill fleas.

Reedmace, or Bulrush as it is still wrongly called, is another plant of pond, ditches and swamps alike. Again it was used as a strewing rush but also in other ways. The pollen produced in profusion by the male part of the flowering mace was used as flour to make sweet creamy biscuits, while the lint of the ripe seeds was used in all sorts of medical and cosmetic ways; when soaked with dew it made the world's first organic wet-wipe.

Gipsywort is one of those plants which pops up in all sorts of damp places from the muddy edges of rivers and ponds to the margins of Willow scrub and damp woodland. Legend has it that would-be gypsies used to dye their skin with extracts of this plant in an attempt to make themselves look more authentic. It would thus appear that there have always been enough fakes across the centuries to give real gypsies a bad name. This has been to the detriment of the cause of herbal medicine as the true wandering people of Eurasia have been good custodians of both prescriptions and herbal practice across the centuries.

Gipsywort does, however, produce a good black dye which stays fast on skin and cloth alike. It also contains an alkaloid which has the ability to affect the activity of iodine in the human body in cases of thyroid deficiency.

The Mints are not confined to watery places but the Peppermint, being a lucky hybrid between our native Watermint and the Spearmint of mint-sauce fame, an early introduction into this country, often grows with its roots in the wet. The hybrid was first recorded in Britain sometimes in the late seventeenth century and rapidly became

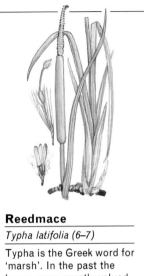

Reedmace

Typha latifolia (6–7)

Typha is the Greek word for 'marsh'. In the past the leaves were greatly valued for thatching, matting, upholstering and caulking wooden ships and barrels. Today the living roots are of great importance in treating waste water.

Gipsywort

Lycopus europaeus (7–9)

Perhaps because of its habitat and its links with the vagabond gypsies, the plant was not used in the past except as a source of dye. Only in the past 100 years has its antibiotic action been discovered and investigated. **CONTAINS** bitters, essential oil, heterosides and tannins.

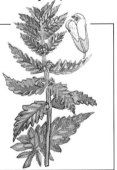

Spearmint
(1) Mentha spicata (8–9)

Watermint
Mentha aquatica (7–10)

Peppermint
(1) Mentha × piperita (7–10)

If you say you don't believe in herbal remedies, next time you reach for that Polo or menthol-tasting sweet, suck it and see how much better you feel. Used since earliest times in Egyptian, Islamic and Hebrew medicine.
CONTAIN essential oils and tannins which react together; Peppermint contains much menthol, Watermint none;
USES: *C:* a simple infusion of the leaves helps you sleep, calms the nerves, for cramps, dizziness, coughs, migraines and flatulence;
 HER: we take it in medicine, sweets and liqueurs such as Pernod and Ouzo, also in sauces and syrups. In large quantities it is said to be aphrodisiac, perhaps that's why the After Eights go so quickly.

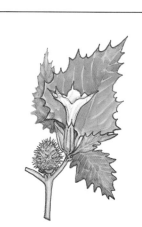

Thorn-apple
(Poison ×××××) Datura stramonium (7–10)

Originally from Central America, it was brought to the Mediterranean and then let loose in Europe and eventually in America. The green conker-like apples placed in surgical spirit produce a mystical green fluorescence but handle with care for it is very poisonous.
CONTAINS the alkaloids hyoscyamine, atropine and scopolamine;
USES: *C:* magical uses;
 HER: salves for scalds and burns, and in the treatment of ulcers and tumours, epilepsy, tetanus and relief of extreme pain.

the favourite mint to use to flavour pastilles and sweets, with or without a hole in the centre. The supply of mint from the wild soon fell behind demand and so large fields were turned over to mint cultivation, the most famous being at Mitcham just outside London.

THORN-APPLES

Summer droughts are not a new phenomenon, although hosepipe bans are a new invention for in these days of washing and washing-up machines, flush loos and the like, each one of us uses more than his or her fair share of water, especially in the drier south-east of England. Village ponds, which traditionally did their best to keep our thirsty Shires well-watered, have always been liable to dry up. When they do, one strange plant is wont to pop up on the muddy scene. The Thorn-apple is a once-seen, never-to-be-forgotten plant with its large white trumpet-shaped flowers dangling down before being replaced by spiky conker-like fruits. It was originally introduced to

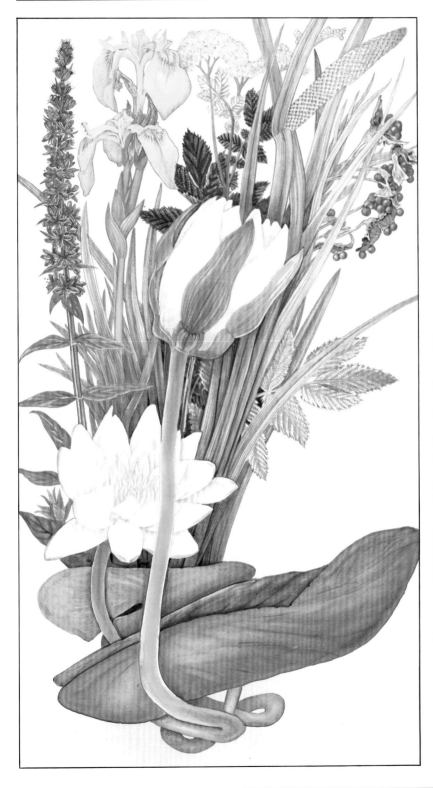

Meandering Rivers and Fenland

1 White Water-lily, *Nymphaea alba*
2 Purple Loosestrife, *Lythrum salicaria*
3 Yellow Flag, *Iris pseudacorus*
4 Meadowsweet, *Filipendula ulmaria*
5 Sweet Flag, *Acorus calamus*
6 Stinking Iris, *Iris foetidissima*

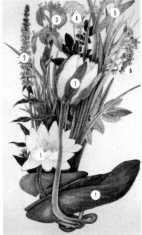

Britain, probably from Turkey, almost at the end of the sixteenth century. It was then taken to America, either by accident or for use as a medicinal plant, where it ran wild as the infamous James Town or Jimpson Weed, killing cattle and people. It is a viciously poisonous plant which, like so many of the other members of the Deadly Nightshade Family, contains a coven of narcotic alkaloids. It was used in witches' brews, producing the sensation of flying through the air, temporary madness and death.

Yet in the hands of science it has found much use in pain-killing and antispasmodic (anti-fit) preparations; and research goes on into its 'truth drug' properties.

We move from this Devil's-apple in good company of the two Angelicas – small and large; these are members of the Carrot Flower Family which pop up in all sorts of damp places, from the edges of ponds to wet woodlands and damp rockscapes down towards the sea.

BESIDE THE SEA

As water, sweetened and made pure again in its passage through the countryside, becomes tainted with tidal salt, the pattern of watery life changes. Reedmace is one of the few plants which make it into those semi-brackish pools which used to typify the natural estuary and shore line before pollution and drainage became widespread.

Likewise, Bladderwrack, that prolific brown seaweed with its own twin floaters, poppers that must be popped, is borne up on the tide to be stranded in beds of Sea Campion. Bladderwrack has long been used as a cure for obesity and certainly, like so many other real weeds

---

Angelica

(1) Angelica sylvestris (7–9)

Archangelica

Angelica archangelica (7–10)

Plants of heavenly origin.
CONTAIN essential oils and coumarin;
USES: restorative and pick-you-up. The latter plant which is not a native once grew in abundance around the Tower of London and in Lincoln's Inn Fields. One Robert Buckeley writing in 1641 suggests that the plant is helpful in extreme labour and when women have been left for dead. It is this plant whose young stems give us candied peel for Christmas cakes;
HER: arthritis, rheumatism and skin disorders.

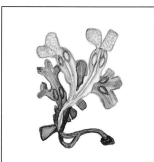

Bladderwrack

Fucus vesiculosus (3–5)

CONTAINS alginates, organic acids and minerals including iodine;
USES: the classic organic soil conditioner of the lazy bed method of permaculture (a specialised method of organic gardening) which kept acidity at bay over the centuries in the wet Celtic climes;
HER: weight watchers – as a source of iodine and stimulant for action of the thyroid.

of the sea, it contains iodine which is now known to stimulate the thyroid and so works wonders in weight-watching circles. It is once again on sale in chemist shops of high repute.

The same cannot be said of the young shoots of sea campion, of which Gerard wrote 'when boiled make an excellent vegetable that ought to be improved for the garden'. I can find no evidence that anyone bothered.

Our coastlines do however provide us with health-giving vegetables and with many plants which, like Brooklime and Watercress, have followed us down the river. The Scurvy-grasses are there in abundance waiting, as they did for the sailors of every ship close beside the docks, full of vitamin C. So, too, we find the Wild Cabbage and Seakale, ancestors of those dreaded 'greens' which we were all urged to eat up and not for the first time either; the phrase *crambi repitita*, which means 'Cabbage warmed up', crops up in ancient Roman scripts and signifies endless repetition – tell me the old old story. The knowledge of these healing plants has been passed down the ages, helping that all-important relationship between healer and healed, together putting the chemical virtues of each plant to good use.

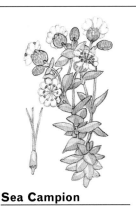

Sea Campion

Silene maritima (6–8)

The word Campion comes from the Latin '*campus*', the field in which the flowers grow, or from 'champion' for the flowers were used to garland the winners in public games.
CONTAINS sugars, essential oil and minerals;
USES: *C:* bladder and stomach complaints, as suggested by the inflated bases of the flowers.

Scurvy-grass

(2) Cochlearia officinalis (5–8)

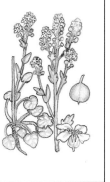

CONTAINS vitamins, bitters, tannins and a glycoside;
USES: *C:* anti-scurvy, mouthwash and diuretic. Perhaps a description of scurvy from Gerard will remind us of the importance of antiscorbutics containing vitamin C in our diet. 'This filthie, lothsome disease, in which the gums are loosed, swolne and exulcerate, the mouth is greevously stinking, the thighes and legs are withall verie often full of bleuspots, and the feete swolne as in dropsie.' If that's enough to put you off, then drink up your orange juice, as the prople of London did their Scurvy-grass drink back in the 1650s.

How else could such an unprepossessing and prickly customer as the Sea Holly or *Eyringium* ever have come into use? The hurtful labour of pulling up this stiff spiny member of the Carrot Family to obtain its roots must have had its just rewards or it would have been left well alone. Yet we find Gerard willing us, well at least some of us, to try candied Sea Holly, 'Good for those that have no delight or

Wild Cabbage
(3) Brassica oleracea (5–8)

Wild Kale
Crambe maritima (6–8)

Pliny praised both the Wild Cabbage and the many cultivated forms then on sale in the markets as a complete do-it-yourself pharmacopoeia, curing everything from dim eyes to drunkenness. In Gerard's words, 'they saye that the brothe wherein the herbe hath been sodden is marvellous good for the sinewes and joints, and likewise for the canker in the eies, called in Greek "Carcinomata", which cannot be cured by any other means, if they be washed therwith.'

Of Kale, much the same could be claimed with the added benefit that the original cultivars came from the coast of Britain. Introduced into our gardens and pharmacies in the late eighteenth century, the true British greens have been doing their bit for a long time.

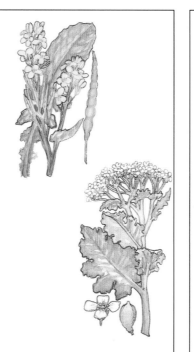

Sea Holly
(10) Eryngium maritimum (7–8)

Gerard tells us 'the roots condited or preserved with sugar are exceeding good to be given to the old and aged people that are consumed and withered with age and which want natural moisture'.
CONTAINS soaps and minerals;
USES: *C/HER:* sweetmeats, 'kissing comfits' to sweeten the breath, dropsy, jaundice, urinary complaints, ear drops and insect stings.

appetite for venery – nourishing and restoring the aged and amending the defects of nature in the younger'. Sea Hollies were in great demand in London, imported from their main centre of re-production in the estuaries around Colchester from the late sixteenth to the middle of the nineteenth century. Virtue or vice, naughty but nice.

COMMON NAMES

Another seaside plant often found growing alongside Sea Holly is the Yellow Horned Poppy or Squatmore: squat meant bruise and so squatmore meant bruiseroot. In no less a publication than the

Yellow Horned Poppy
Glaucium flavum (6–9)

Glaucus was the name of a fisherman who leaped into the sea and 'by transmutation strange' became a Sea God. A plant of witches and used more as a charm than in medicine, it was thought to induce madness.

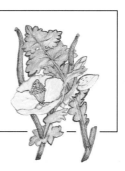

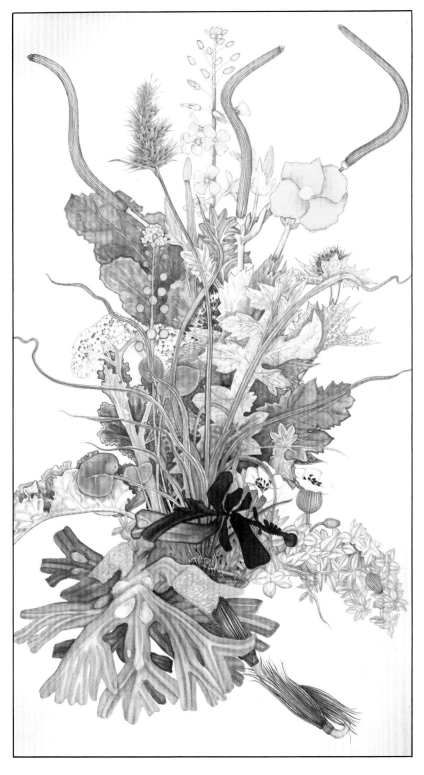

The Margins of the Sea

1 Bladderwrack, *Fucus vesiculosus*
2 Scurvy-grass, *Cochlearia officinalis*
3 Wild Kale, *Crambe maritima*
4 Yellow Horned Poppy, *Glaucium flavum*
5 Sand Sedge, *Carex arenaria*
6 Wild Cabbage, *Brassica oleracea*
7 Sea Holly, *Eryngium maritimum*
8 Sea Campion, *Silene maritima*

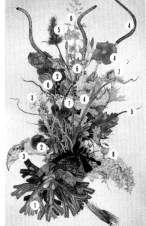

Philosophical Transactions of the Royal Society of 1698 we find the following account of this handsome plant:

> A certain person made a pye of the roots of this plant, supposing them to be the roots of the Eryngo [Sea Holly], of which he had before eaten pyes, which were very pleasant, and eating it while it was hot, became delerious, and having voided a stool in a white chamber pot, fancied it to be gold, breaking the pot to pieces, and desiring what he imagined to be gold might be preserved as such. Also his man and his maid servant eating of the same pye, fancied of what they saw to be gold.

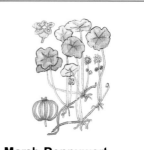

Marsh Pennywort

(1) Hydrocotyle vulgaris (6–8)

CONTAINS soaps, essential oils and tannins; **USES:** *C/HER:* purge, vomit and diuretic. The larger Asiatic species was imported into Britain as a very powerful diuretic to shift large quantities of urine out of the body, relieving strain on the heart. *R:* continues on both species.

Two new common or vulgar names spring to mind, Stools Gold or Mind-your-own-Business, perhaps reminding us why so many of these ancient cures fell into disrepute, taking others more worthy of investigation with them.

One such plant has indeed followed us all the way from mountain tarn to brackish dyke and that is the Marsh Pennywort or White Rot. Mistakenly vilified by shepherds for rotting the livers of their sheep, as were many other plants of the marshy places in which the larvae of the real culprit, the liverfluke, thrived, Marsh Pennywort was used to break the stone and cleanse the urine of the painful gravels. This shy little water plant, whose tiny flowers oft go unnoticed, is now being researched as a cure for both tuberculosis and leprosy; diseases which are still the scourge of the developing world, many of whose people cannot afford costly modern drugs. Tuberculosis in a new form which is immune to modern antibiotics is now sweeping parts of the rich world. Perhaps here is real reason for another change of name, pennywort may yet be revalued to become Mark- or even Yen-wort.

THE EVER-CHANGING SCENE

Over the centuries our watery landscapes have changed out of all recognition. As time wore on after the last Ice Age, the rich supplies of minerals released from the crushed rock were gradually used up, and the growth of wetland plants and that process of paludification slowed the flow of water through our lakes and river systems. Large areas of our wetlands became cut off from the effects of flowing water

Sand Sedge

Carex arenaria (6–7)

A common plant of the seaside where it 'stitches' the sand together and helps to initiate the formation of dunes, nature's own coastal defences. This is the only one of our sedges which has been widely used in herbal medicine. It has been used as a substitute for the American import sarsaparilla, a spring-time tonic.

CONTAINS soaps, tannins and essential oil and resin;
USES: *HER:* rheumatic pains, bronchitis and as a diuretic.

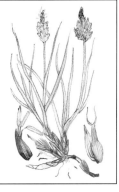

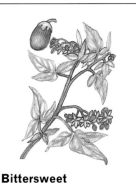

Bittersweet

(1) (Poison ××××) Solanum dulcamara (6–9)

A bitter plant with a sweet aftertaste but do not try for it is very poisonous. Solanum comes from the Latin word for 'solace'.
CONTAINS alkaloids, glycosides, sugars, soaps and resins;
USES: *C:* treats wounds, as a sedative and pain reliever;
 HER: bronchitis, asthma, eczema;
 HOM: psoriasis, eczema, nervous paralysis, cystitis and rheumatism.

and so began to go sour and acid. This provided ideal conditions for the growth and spread of the Bog Mosses, the Sphagna. So from our estuaries to the flanks of our highest mountains, bogs began to develop, the layers of acid peat getting thicker and thicker by the year.

The people of the New Stone Age certainly helped the process along. Their relentless cycle of slash-and-burn agriculture left the soil bare and open to erosion and leaching by rain. They knew nothing of the use of fertilisers and agricultural lime so the soil became more impoverished and more acid. The trees could no longer regenerate and grow, and large areas of landscape were in a state of terminal collapse. Then something very magical took place: enormous blankets of peat began to cover the terrain, healing our mountains and lowlands, especially in the wetter west.

Landscapes which had for thousands of years been covered with mixed forest opened up and became the wet bogs, heaths and moorlands we know today. Trees were replaced by low-growing plants which could tolerate the acid, mineral-poor conditions, their only new supplies of nutrients coming from the rain which fell directly on the surface of the peat. Rain in its natural state is slightly acid, almost pure soft water; great for washing your hair but not for keeping vegetation supplied with the minerals it needs. Some plants of the old regime, such as Bittersweet and Remote Flowered Sedge, hung on, but eventually the Bog Mosses took over.

HEALING MOSSES

Bog Mosses are truly amazing plants. Each one acts like a tiny growing sponge; massed together they form hummocks which soak up the rain, keeping the surface saturated, alive and always growing upwards. Each one holds many times its own weight of water; dried they make ideal nappies and absorbent wound dressings and have been used as such for centuries.

During the First World War when the terrible wounds inflicted on the men in the trenches had to be dealt with, the collection of Bog Moss from our hills became an important part of the war effort. Shiploads were sent across from the swamps and bogs of Canada; even the strict Presbyterian ministers of the Scottish Highlands and Islands allowed their parishioners to glean the healing mosses from the hills on Sundays; while the great shooting estates opened up their lodges as centres of collection, drying and distribution.

Another group of plants which provided organic dressings and wet-wipes, though on a lesser scale, was the Bog Cottons whose heads of white linted fruits cover the boglands like snow in summer. These also provide the hardy upland sheep with the so-called 'early bite', the first fresh food of the year.

Two other plants which thrive on the acid peatland each tell a different story. Bog Asphodel, a member of the Lily Flower Family, turns the bogscapes first green with its sword-shaped leaves, then yellow with its flowers, and finally a vinous orange thanks to its erect spikes of fruits. Shepherds always feared this plant for they knew that it gave their sheep the dreaded rickets. Scientists pooh-poohed the idea, saying that it was the acid grazing which provided little or no bone-strengthening calcium that was to blame. Modern research has shown the locals to be right, for the plant contains natural

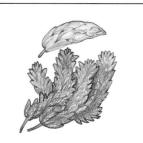

Bog Moss

Sphagnum subsecundum

Widespread across Britain but commoner in the wetter west, being rapidly made rarer thanks to drainage and modern methods of peat cutting. It should not be collected from the wild in Britain but it could be grown sustainably.
CONTAINS cellulose, acids and pigments;
USES: makes excellent absorptive, antiseptic medical wipes and nappies;
C/HER: wound dressings.

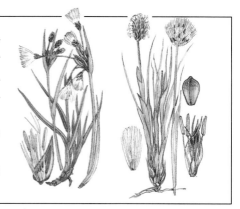

Common Cotton-grass

Eriophorum angustifolium (6)

Bog Cotton

Eriophorum vaginatum (4–5)

Members of the Sedge Family, the former can grow in both bogs and poor fens where there is some water movement and mineral enrichment. The latter thrives in the most acid bogland habitats.

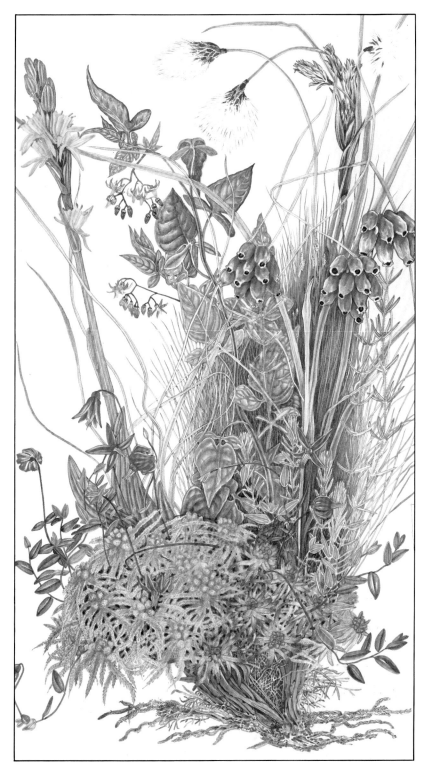

Acid Bogland

1 Cranberry, *Vaccinium oxycoccus*
2 Bog Asphodel, *Narthecium ossifragum*
3 Bittersweet, *Solanum dulcamara*
4 Bog Cotton, *Eriophorum vaginatum*
5 Remote Sedge, *Carex remota*
6 Common Cotton-grass, *Eriophorum angustifolium*
7 Cross-leaved Heath, *Erica tetralix*
8 Bog Moss, *Sphagnum fimbriatum*
9 Bog Moss, *Sphagnum capillifolium*

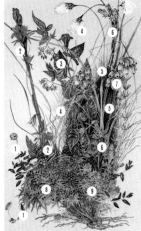

chemicals which inhibit the manufacture of the all-important vitamin D. The flowers were, however, used as a substitute for Saffron, both in cooking and in medicine,

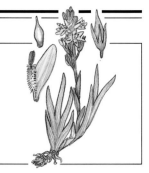

Bog Asphodel

(Poison ××) Narthecium ossifragum (7–9)

Asphodels were to the Greeks the flowers of death for they grew in Hades.
CONTAINS soaps, pigments and glycoside;
USES: in the Middle Ages as a dye; and the root as 'food for a king'.

and provided a yellow hair-dye into the bargain.

Cranberry is not as easy to find for it creeps across the surface of the bog maintaining a low profile, out of the way of the drying wind of winter. Its tiny but perfect pink flowers are well worth looking at under a magnifying glass; each one is like the head of a crane complete with beak. The round red-black succulent fruits are also worth searching for; they are a good source of vitamin C, best eaten after the first frosts of autumn or even in the following spring.

Its larger cousin, found on the peatlands of the maritime states of what is now America, is today grown commercially for export across the world. The Pilgrim Fathers soon learned of the importance of this plant in the diet and cuisine of the local Wampanoag Indians who used it as part of their famous marching rations, pemmican, a dried cake of meat and fat. The Pilgrim Fathers adapted it as the sauce which went with the turkey on Thanksgiving Day and it was quickly exported to England, a 'unique' product of the New World territories. Our own Cranberry was, of course, already in use in sauces, pies and puddings, for it was much more common and abundant before mass drainage became the order of the day.

PEAT AND PEAT BATHS

Acid peat, though mainly made of the bog mosses, contains the partially decayed remains of all the other sorts of plants which make up the bogland flora. It is therefore a unique product containing all of the chemicals, celluloses, phenols, anthracenes, tannins and resins, and their breakdown products in its make-up. On the continent of Europe, especially in Czechoslovakia, Germany and Poland, peat is used in spa towns and medical institutes to treat patients suffering from diseases and conditions ranging from stress, rheumatism and

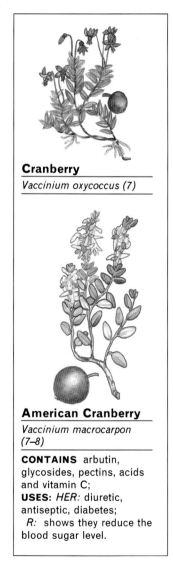

Cranberry
Vaccinium oxycoccus (7)

American Cranberry
Vaccinium macrocarpon (7–8)

CONTAINS arbutin, glycosides, pectins, acids and vitamin C;
USES: *HER:* diuretic, antiseptic, diabetes;
R: shows they reduce the blood sugar level.

arthritis to skin cancer. The main method of application is immersion in peat baths, with or without the addition of other herbal extracts. Such techniques were pioneered in Sri Lanka and India; and the North American Indians used hot bath and sauna-type therapies with added herbs to treat a similar range of complaints. Baths and aromatherapy are now becoming popular in Britain with very positive results, so much so that the latter is even becoming accepted as part of a NHS prescription.

THE 'FEVERED' PLANET

Today the wetlands of Britain and of the world are under massive attack. They are being drained and drenched with insecticide in an attempt to control malaria because the mosquitoes which transmit the disease from one person to another live in wet watery places. Peat is being dug up for use in horticulture or to be burned in massive power stations to generate energy. Another reason for the mass destruction of this resource is to grow food and cash-crops on the organic peatland soils in an attempt to feed and service the now exploding human population.

Some of the food we eat is turned into heat which keeps our bodies up to working temperature; for a normal healthy person this is 37°C (98.6°F). If our temperature fell a few degrees below that norm we would suffer from hypothermia and soon die. The body fat we store not only helps to insulate our body core from rapid loss of heat but it also acts as an energy store on which our personal life-support system can draw if the need arises.

If our bodies are attacked by disease-producing organisms, bacteria, viruses or the blood parasite which causes malaria, we become fevered. If the attack is not kept under control we overheat and die. Six or seven degrees up and we have little hope of survival, six or seven degrees down and the same is true.

Recent research has shown that the Earth itself is like a gigantic living thing; some talk about a living envelope called the Biosphere, some use the name Gaia. Whatever we call it we now know that the Earth too has a 'normal' temperature, the average temperature of the atmospheric blanket. We also know that the Earth can suffer both from 'hypothermia' and from 'fever'. If the average temperature of the atmospheric blanket falls by six or seven degrees the next ice age will be on the way, covering the high mountains and much more of the northern and southern continents, islands and oceans with glaciers and ice sheets. The now humid tropics would also get much drier and life for us human beings would become much more difficult. Likewise, if the temperature of the Earth rose by six or seven degrees, much of what is left of the glaciers of the last ice age could melt and world sea levels would rise, flooding large areas of our most fertile land and many of our largest cities with salt water.

The Earth, as a habitat for humans and all the other many forms of land life with which we share the planet, is held in a delicate balance. There is now good, or rather very bad, evidence to show that the human population is acting like a disease-producing organism. We, yes you and I, could be causing the temperature of the Earth to rise above normal.

Remember, all living things are made from those invisible gases from the air, and the bulk is made of carbon. We are now destroying forests and other natural vegetation and the soils which supported them at the rate of one hectare every second. We are draining wetlands and peatlands and burning fossil fuels as if there were no tomorrow. All this releases carbon in the form of carbon dioxide into the atmosphere. Carbon dioxide is a greenhouse gas which means it traps and holds the heat rays of the sun, warming up the atmospheric blanket.

The ways in which the normal temperature of both a human 'patient' and the planetary 'patient' is controlled are very complex, and in the case of the latter we are not sure exactly what is going to happen. However, the writing is firmly on the wall that we should now do everything in our power to help cool the Earth down. We must all use energy wisely. We must stop destroying any more of our natural vegetation. We should stop the spread of deserts by planting trees on a massive scale, the right trees in the right places. We should stop drainage of wetlands and exploitation of peatlands and allow them to rehabilitate and grow again, for as they grow they will lock up carbon dioxide in the healing peat blanket, cooling the fevered brow of Planet Earth.

CHAPTER FIVE

People-made and people-managed

At the World Environmental Summit held in Rio de Janeiro in 1992, more than 160 heads of state, prime ministers and the like, signed a directive aimed at protecting biodiversity. In effect they agreed to look after all the different sorts of plants and animals with which we must learn to share this planet. The rights and wrongs of this document will, I am sure, be debated long after the next World Summit, if that ever happens, for biodiversity is not solely an attribute of nature and naturalness, and so it means looking after much more than just our national parks and nature reserves.

When the first British herbalists were seeking their medicines within the almost totally-wooded landscapes of 10,000 years ago, it must have been an arduous process, for neither roads nor biodiversity were commonplace.

As the forests were cleared to make way for cattle and crops, grasslands, shrublands and small woodlots came into being, each flanked by less stable edge or boundary communities in which many different plants and animals could live; and the biodiversity of Britain bloomed. Likewise, as mines, quarries and gravel pits began to scar the land they too opened up new opportunities for the plants and insects of earlier times and pioneer habitats. In fact, today, even a well-managed quarry looks like a piece of late glacial landscape with bare broken rock, gravel, sand, silt and pools of open water, all brimful of mineral promise; providing more space for other living things. Forest clearance meant that some plants which had for millennia been rarities, surviving only in tiny little open areas within the forest and on cliffs and mountain tops, soon became commonplace.

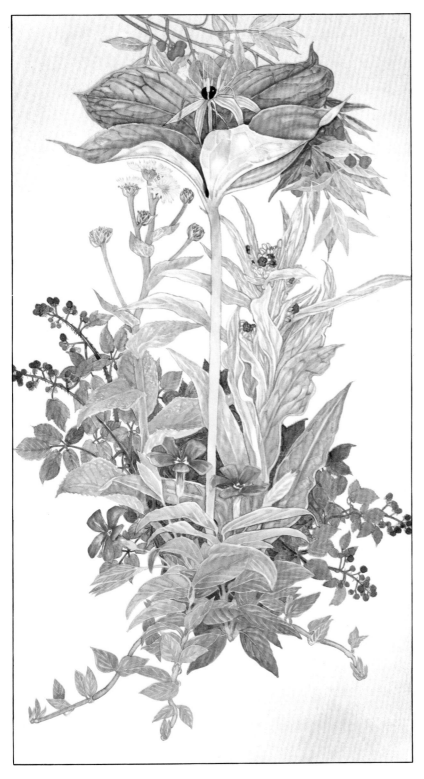

Coppice Woodland – a people managed habitat of great diversity

1 Periwinkle, *Vinca minor*
2 Bramble or Blackberry, *Rubus fruticosus* agg.
3 Elecampane, *Inula helenium*
4 Herb Paris, *Paris quadrifolia*
5 Hound's Tongue, *Cynoglossum officinale*
6 Spindle Tree, *Euonymus europaeus*

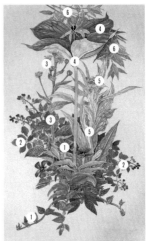

Reduction of forest cover also, of course, led to a reduction of certain types of forest life. Another result was soil erosion and, especially in the wetter west, the leaching and acidification of the soil long before our modern hyperacid rain fell upon the scene.

Similar effects can be seen in just about every temperate country of the world; as people have come to rule the landscape some aspects of biodiversity increased. It is only in comparatively recent times that this people-produced biodiversity has been rapidly replaced by more and more uniformity, thanks to intensive farming, the growing of single crops over large areas and the use of herbicides, pesticides and fertilisers.

It would also appear true that over this latter period, best called the decades of destruction, allergies have become more commonplace among the human population, as have stress-related diseases and the problems relating to an increasing geriatric population, at least in the rich developed world. It is, of course, in these very countries that people are becoming more divorced from those breaths of fresh air, the healing power of their own natural vegetation and the rhythm of the seasons.

WOODLAND MANAGED AS COPPICE

Thanks to the fact that many of our most useful native trees appear to thrive on a regular short-back-and-sides, the art and craft of coppice-management has been developed. Coppicing begins with a single maiden trunk which is cut off before its prime. Each tree then resprouts from suckers or buds around its base to produce a sustainable crop of new stout shoots growing out from each 'coppice stool'. Depending on the amount of time left between each cut, the length and thickness of the shoot will vary, thus providing a range of wood sizes to suit all purposes, including offcuts for firewood and the burnt ash for making soap and glazing pottery. A certain number of trees are left to grow to maturity for use in the local construction industry. From Neolithic times onwards more and more of our woodlands became managed in this way, right up to the time that coal became widely used as fuel, tainting our atmosphere and our countryside with acid rain and smog.

Well-managed coppice woodland consists of a patchwork of plots, each in a different stage of growth, each stage adding to the diversity of local life. At the beginning of each coppice-cycle the ground is flooded with sunlight providing almost grassland conditions. Later in the cycle, these are gradually replaced by ever-deepening shade, ideal for scrubland and woodland plants. In amongst these resprouting coppice stools, some of which are more than 2000, a few even 4000, years of age, our liberated wild flowers could find their own particular eco-niche, a well-managed but ever-changing home. The system worked well for herbalists, who could gather a multitude of varied healing plants in a relatively small area already tamed with roads and tracks. These included markers of ancient woodland such as Yellow Archangel and Herb Paris, backed up by Hound's Tongue and Bramble with introductions such as Elecampane and Blue Periwinkle; a floral prescription for a healthy countryside and healthy people. Coppices were the first well-managed chemist's shops, each one a growing concern.

PLANTS OF THE ANCIENT WOODLAND

Yellow Archangel, blooming at the time of the feast of St Michael, is a close relative of the White Dead-nettle with which it shares its virtues. Both have a disagreeable smell, unless you happen to be a weasel, for both the plants and the animal share the same scent and were said to keep the area free from snakes. Water distilled from the plants was recommended by Gerard, 'to make the heart merrie, to make goode colour in the face and to refresh the vitall spirits'.

A plant with such a strange form as Herb Paris with its four equal leaves and single central flower just had to have singular magical

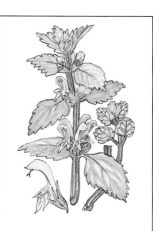

Yellow Archangel

(1) Lamiastrum galeobdolon (5–6)

Said to flower on the feast of St Michael the Archangel. *Lamium* is Latin for 'throat', *galeobdolon* is Greek for the 'smell of a weasel'.
CONTAINS flavones, mucilages and tannins;
USES: along with the much commoner White Dead Nettle;
 HER: infusion of the flower stems for menstrual and menopause problems, also for disorders related to the prostate gland.
 HOM: tincture for catarrh, bronchitis and menstrual problems.

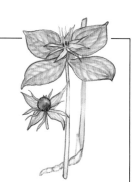

Herb Paris

(Poison ×××) Paris quadrifolia (4–6)

CONTAINS saponins which are toxic, attacking the blood corpuscles;
USES: C: antidote for poisons; with wine for cholic; and specifically used for sores around fingers and toenails;
 HOM: fainting, encephalitis and digestive problems.

Bramble or Blackberry

(3) Rubus fruticosus (6–8)

CONTAINS tannins, organic acids and vitamins;
USES: the fruit yields a dye which is grey on wool
and slate-blue on silk, while the green shoots
provide a black dye;
  C: against snakebites and as a highly valued
mouth and throat gargle, used to fasten loose teeth
at one end and ease piles at the other;
  HER: an anti-diarrhoea syrup of special use for
children is produced from the fruits.

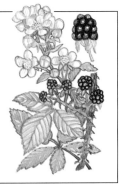

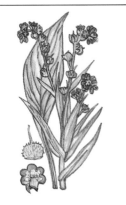

properties. *Par* in Latin means both 'equal' and 'a pair' and so the
plant was used in the divination of pairing or marriage. One complex
ritual demanded that two girls sit in silence throughout the first hour
of a new day. During this time they would remove one hair from their
heads for each year of their lives, laying them beside the plant on a
clean linen cloth. As the clock struck one, the hairs were burned, a
charm was spoken and their future husbands were revealed each to
her own but not to each other.

Hound's Tongue, which likes more open ground, gets its name from
the strange panting blue-pink colour of its flowers. This, together with
its smell of mice, appears to have made it an ideal charm against the
bite of dogs, baldness and diseases of the skin. Despite its Latin name
Cynoglossum it is not a constituent of the infamous Cynoglossal Pills of
Byzantine Medicine, which were really made of minced dogs' tongues.

Bramble can grow in deep shade but flowers and fruits best where
there is at least dappled sunlight. A blessed plant in Scotland, where
few other fruits ripen in the short cool summers, it is today the
commonest fruit of our countryside. Bramble is also our natural
gleaner, its thorns plucking wool from the backs of passing sheep
ready to be used as
medical swabs or for
spinning. The Spindle Tree,
another shrub which does
well in the coppice cycle,
provided the wood to make
the spindles. Its strange
orange-red fruits shaped

Hound's Tongue

*(Poison ××) Cynoglossum
officinale (5–9)*

CONTAINS alkaloids
including cynoglossine,
which is toxic to cold-
blooded animals but not to
mammals, and tannins;
USES: *C:* bite of mad dogs,
baldness and burns;
  HER: sores, skin diseases
and piles;
  HOM: skin disorders.

Spindle Tree

(Poison ×××) Euonymus europaeus (5–6)

CONTAINS bitters, cardiotonics, the fruit is
rich in pigments;
USES: spindles, skewers, musical instruments
and artists' charcoal;
  C: as an insecticide of great use against lice;
  HER: diuretic, purgative and to aid digestion.

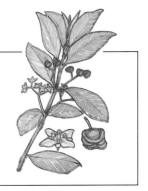

like a priest's biretta contain a complex of poisons which speed up the contraction rate of the intestine and so should be left well alone. Aptly named *Euonymus* after the mother of the Furies, it was said to warn of plague if it flowered early in May rather than in June. At such a time a herbalist may well have made sure that Elecampane was close at hand.

PLANTS INTRODUCED FROM ABROAD WHICH HAVE MADE THEMSELVES AT HOME

Elecampane, or Wild Sunflower, a more descriptive though less apt name as it is not truly wild, is today widespread but still a rarity in Britain. It was introduced from Asia via Europe and must have been grown widely in gardens from which it has escaped into the wild. The reasons for its popularity are given in John Pechey's *Compleat Herbal* published in 1694.

> The fresh Root being candied, or dried, and powder'd, mix'd with Hony or Sugar, is very good in a Difficulty of Breath'ng, Asthma, and an old Cough. Being taken after supper, it helps Concoction. It is also commended as an excellent preservative against the Plague. Being taken in the Morning, it forces Urine and the Courses. Half a pint of White-wine, wherein the slic'd Roots have been infus'd three Days, taken in the morning fasting, cures the Green-sickness. A Decoction of the Root, taken inwardly, or outwardly applied, is commended by some for Convulsions, Contusions, and the Hip-Gout. The Roots boyl'd in Wine, or the fresh Juice infus'd in it, and drunk, kills and expels Worms. Wine that is every where prepar'd with this Root in *Germany*, and often drunk, wonderfully quickens the sight.

The Little Blue Periwinkle is probably a native plant and this shy though rampaging shade plant is today widespread in our woodlands. Used to decorate graves in the past and to garland heroic criminals on their way to the gallows or worse, it is a plant long associated with death yet it is included in many love potions.

A manuscript from the fourteenth century advises, 'Periwinkle powdered with Earthworms eaten together by husband and wife

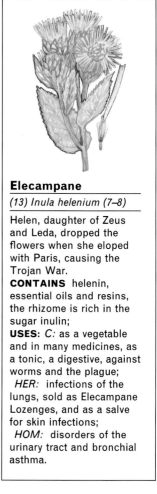

Elecampane

(13) Inula helenium (7–8)

Helen, daughter of Zeus and Leda, dropped the flowers when she eloped with Paris, causing the Trojan War.
CONTAINS helenin, essential oils and resins, the rhizome is rich in the sugar inulin;
USES: *C:* as a vegetable and in many medicines, as a tonic, a digestive, against worms and the plague;
HER: infections of the lungs, sold as Elecampane Lozenges, and as a salve for skin infections;
HOM: disorders of the urinary tract and bronchial asthma.

invokes love between them.' It is a member of the flower family to which it gives its name, a family which, thanks to the Rosy Periwinkle of Madagascar, has given a desperate modern world chemical substances now helping to cure childhood leukaemia and Hodgkin's disease, two forms of cancer. Our plant is now being researched for similar hidden virtues; some indication of success has been signalled in the case of Alzheimer's disease. The world lives in hope for, despite its other name of senile dementia, this is a disease which can strike both young and old. We should perhaps be heartened by the knowledge that the white-flowered form of our plant has long been regarded as the symbol of the 'pleasure of memory'. Take a close look at the flower which has great internal beauty and remember the native woodlands of all our pasts are also woodlands which hold so much hope for all our futures.

HEDGEROWS

Although most of our hedgerows were planted in the not too far distant past they soon became extensions of what was left of our native woodlands: pleached and espaliered shrubberies and double herbaceous borders, complete with high-rise homes at regular intervals where trees were left to grow. These standard trees were a source of sustainable timber ready for use on the farm.

In places, these hedgerows were the only natural tall structures and became highways of landscape and biodiversity over large areas of Britain. That was until the mania of ripping out the hedgerows began in the post-war years. During the last five decades of destruction

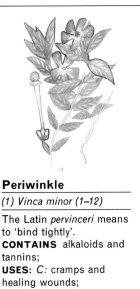

Periwinkle

(1) Vinca minor (1–12)

The Latin *pervinceri* means to 'bind tightly'.
CONTAINS alkaloids and tannins;
USES: *C:* cramps and healing wounds;
 HER: intestinal complaints, skin diseases especially of the scalp, uterine haemorrhages and other internal bleeding;
 R: active, ongoing on the alkaloids.

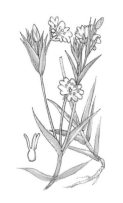

Greater Stitchwort

Stellaria holostea (6–9)

Known as 'All Bones' for it is so brittle that its root can never be pulled up.
CONTAINS soaps and minerals;
USES: *HER:* as an antidote to stitch.

Agrimony

(14) Agrimonia eupatoria (6–9)

Mithridates Eupator, a Pontine Emperor, was an expert in herbal therapy.
CONTAINS tannins and an essential oil;
USES: *C:* to remove cataracts and for other eye complaints, wounds, warts and snakebites;
 HER: to purify the blood, liver tonic, freshens the breath, counteracts stomach acidity, eyewash and to induce sleep; Bach.

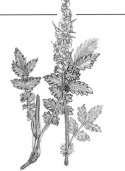

almost 200,000 miles of
hedgerow habitat have
been destroyed, so
alienating both people and
nature from their woodland
roots.

Greater Stitchwort,
Agrimony, Herb Robert
and Lords-and-Ladies are
perhaps our best known
hedge-bottom plants; while

Herb Robert

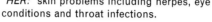

(3) Geranium robertianum (4–7)

The *Ortus Sanitatus*, the standard herbal for
hundreds of years, was written for Robert,
Duke of Normandy, in 1490. The plant either
took its name from him or from a less down-
to-earth character, Robin Goodfellow.
CONTAINS bitters, tannins and an essential
oil;
USES: *C:* wounds, ulcers, piles and kidney
infections;
 HER: skin problems including herpes, eye
conditions and throat infections.

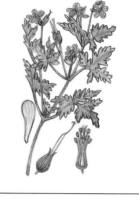

Dog Roses, red, white and every shade between, were just part of the
barbed brigade of thorny shrubs which made our hedges the self-
repairing impenetrable barriers they were: growing guardians of our
dwindling wildlife heritage.

Agrimony, reputedly used to clear eyes by removing film from their
surface, is the Egremoine mentioned by Chaucer who recommended
its use for 'alle woundes and bad back', and Gerard used a decoction
of its leaves 'for them that have naughty livers'.

Greater Stitchwort goes under at least 100 common names, most
of which relate to the Devil and to evil things; its swollen stems remind
people of finger-bones reaching up from the grave. It was used to
relieve pain caused by overexertion and was gathered only on the day
of rest, and so was called White Sunday.

Herb Robert is another plant with 100 common names or more,
most of them not relating to the Devil but to Robin Goodfellow, Tom
Thumb or other mischievous fairy-like characters. Its other names
such as Cuckoo's Eye and Cuckoo Meat link the plant with the coming
of spring, the revels of early summer and with sex; this gave both
Gerard and Culpeper reason for labelling it as 'an Herb of Venus
despite the fact that it carries a man's name'.

So, too, with Cuckoo Pint or Lords-and-Ladies which has more
names than either of the above: names which include one of the
longest, Kitty-come-down-the-lane-jump-up-and-kiss-me, and some of
the commonest, Parson's Billycock, Priest's Pintle, Dog's Dibble and
just plain Cuckoo Cock. Take your pick or make up your own for this
member of the Arum Flower Family.

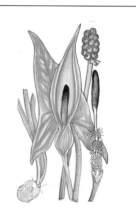

Cuckoo Pint

*(Poison ×××) Arum
maculatum (4–5)*

CONTAINS a bitter
compound called aroine
which is toxic, attacking the
nervous system, it can also
cause blisters.
USES: starch, the rhizome
can be eaten but must be
cooked well;
 C: to draw poison from
wounds and ulcers;
 HER: plague, polyps of
the nose, coughs and loss
of appetite;
 HOM: bronchial catarrh,
whooping cough and
bronchitis.

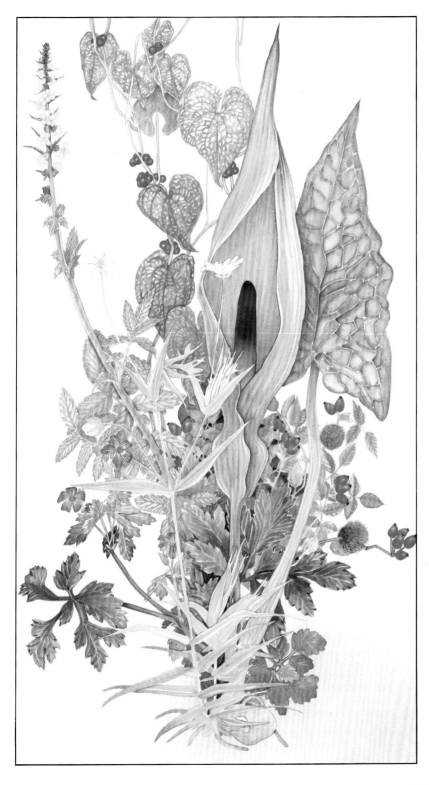

Hedgerows – natural highways of diversity

1 Herb Robert, *Geranium robertianum*
2 Agrimony, *Agrimonia eupatoria*
3 Greater Stitchwort, *Stellaria holostea*
4 Black Bryony, *Tamus communis*
5 Cuckoo Pint, *Arum maculatum*
6 Dog Rose, *Rosa canina*

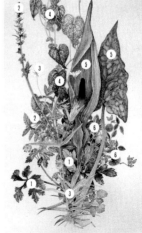

Its roots, along with those of the Early Purple Orchid, were a constituent of that strengthening food salep. Those grown in the fallow fields around Portland and sold under the name of Portland Sago were especially recommended because they had the taste of arrowroot. The strengthening power of the starch extracted from the Portland rootstocks was once in great demand. In Elizabethan times it was the only starch which could stiffen the enormous lawn neck-ruffs designed by the haute couturiers and worn by the followers of fashion. This was despite the havoc it wreaked on the skins of the hands of the laundry maids who put the starch around the necks of the ladies of the wardrobe of Good Queen Bess. It was perhaps partly because of this that the Queen eventually commanded men to stand at the gates of London to cut down all ruffs more than a yard deep.

Dog Roses were among the first of our wild plants to be brought to heel by horticulture; selection and breeding adding to their already immense diversity and to the lasting quality of their flowers. The name 'dog' dates back perhaps to Pliny, for he recorded that a member of the Pretorian Guard after being bitten by a mad dog used a root of the plant to cure himself of hydrophobia. Wild Roses are often covered with strange growths called galls produced in response to certain insects laying their eggs within the tissues of the plant. One called Robin's Pincushion is the nursery within which the next generation of a gall wasp develops, together with the assorted larvae of other insects, predators and parasites. The dried galls, insects and all, used to be collected and sold as powdered Briar balls or bedeguars to cure a number of ailments. Rose-hips are a good source of a really effective itching powder, the hairy seeds within; while the coloured hips are rich in vitamins, especially A and P, and were used as Gerard tells us 'for makeing the most pleasante meales and banketting dishes or tartes'.

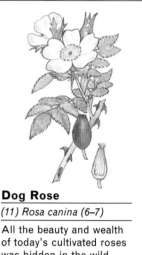

Dog Rose

(11) Rosa canina (6–7)

All the beauty and wealth of today's cultivated roses was hidden in the wild varieties until released and put on show by centuries of selection and breeding. **CONTAINS** vitamins C, P, and protovitamin A (a rich source in the fruit), essential oils, pigments and tannins;
USES: perfumery;
 C: dog bites, hydrophobia;
 HER: gall bladder and kidney complaints, diuretic and anti-diarrhoea. Rosehip syrup is an excellent tonic and stimulant; Bach.

Black Bryony

(Poison ××××) Tamus communis (5–7)

A member of the Yam Flower Family, the family which gave the world one of its most important plants – the Mexican Yam – source of the active element of the oral contraceptive.
CONTAINS diosgenene, a poisonous alkaloid, a histamine-like substance and calcium oxalate;
USES: *HER:* treating bruises (its French name is the 'Battered Wife Plant') although its use has dangers;
 HOM: a tincture is used against sunstroke.

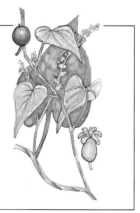

ROADSIDES

Like hedges, many roadside verges are a recent addition to our countryside but some do date back to Roman times; while drovers' tracks and even corduroy-like roads of logs found preserved in the peat bogs are from even earlier periods. Road margins, enriched by manure, dust and seeds carried on or within passing people and animals, are now home to a great diversity of plants. Members of the Carrot Flower Family often dominate the scene with their predominantly white cartwheel heads of flowers. Fool's Parsley is commonest in the south, replaced in part by Sweet Cicely further north. The former is not a very nice plant and has been avoided over the centuries, while the latter with its aniseed-scented flowers and large black seed pods always found more favour. Used as a salad herb – its roots boiled with oil were eaten – it is also one of the bouquet of herbs used to put the flavour into Chartreuse; and used in powdered form it makes a condiment for puddings, especially fresh Strawberries.

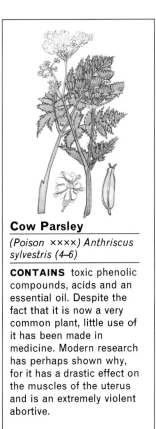

Cow Parsley

(Poison ××××) Anthriscus sylvestris (4–6)

CONTAINS toxic phenolic compounds, acids and an essential oil. Despite the fact that it is now a very common plant, little use of it has been made in medicine. Modern research has perhaps shown why, for it has a drastic effect on the muscles of the uterus and is an extremely violent abortive.

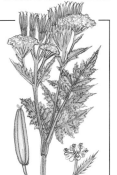

Sweet Cicely

Myrrhis odorata (6–7)

CONTAINS an essential oil which includes anethol, giving it the fragrance of aniseed;
USES: pot herb, vegetable, and mixed with wax to make a fragrant furniture polish;
 HER: tonic, diuretic, also to lower the blood pressure;
 R: anethol stimulates all glands, increasing the flow of saliva, digestive juices and milk.

Culpeper used candied Sweet Cicely roots to ward off plague, while Gerard considered 'the roots boiled with oil and vinegar ... are good for old people who are dull and without courage, rejoicing and comforting the heart, and increasing their lust and strength'. The true aniseed essence comes from *Pimpinella anisum*, a Mediterranean plant, the oil from the seeds of which contains 90 per cent anethol, one of the best natural carminatives (treatment for flatulence) known to medicine.

However, have a care, mistakes in identification could prove fatal, and again, remember the warning at the beginning of this book,

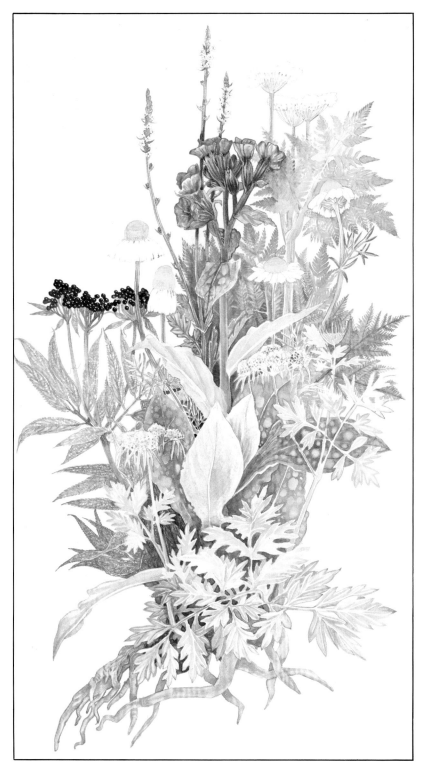

Roadside Verges – linear nature reserves

1 Dwarf Elder, *Sambucus ebulus*
2 Wild Chamomile, *Matricaria recutita*
3 Vervain, *Verbena officinalis*
4 Lungwort, *Pulmonaria officinalis*
5 Sweet Cicely, *Myrrhis odorata*
6 Fool's Parsley, *Aethusa cynapium*

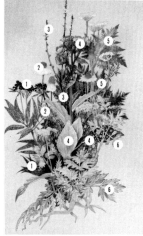

Leave wild flowers (even common ones) for others to enjoy. If you really want to use them, buy seed and grow them in your garden.

Dwarf Elder or Danewort, though not a member of the same family, does produce similar cartwheels of white flowers. It is much commoner on the Continent than here in Britain where it is often found associated, at least in legend, with the sites of past battles with the Danes. Its specific name is *ebulus*, meaning to bubble up from the blood of our enemies, and as if to prove it much of the plant turns red in autumn, a red which stains the ground beneath with the black of dried blood. The whole plant then disappears without trace until the following spring. To bring the illusion down to earth, danes also means diarrhoea and in Latin signifies an unpleasant smell for, like its larger brother which has been called God's Stinking Tree, it also emanates a nasty aroma.

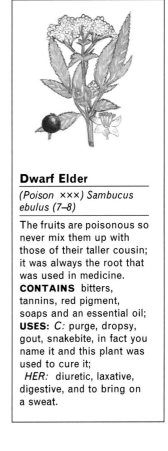

Dwarf Elder

(Poison ×××) Sambucus ebulus (7–8)

The fruits are poisonous so never mix them up with those of their taller cousin; it was always the root that was used in medicine.
CONTAINS bitters, tannins, red pigment, soaps and an essential oil;
USES: *C:* purge, dropsy, gout, snakebite, in fact you name it and this plant was used to cure it;
  HER: diuretic, laxative, digestive, and to bring on a sweat.

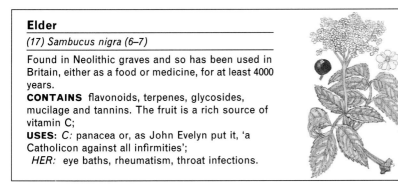

Elder

(17) Sambucus nigra (6–7)

Found in Neolithic graves and so has been used in Britain, either as a food or medicine, for at least 4000 years.
CONTAINS flavonoids, terpenes, glycosides, mucilage and tannins. The fruit is a rich source of vitamin C;
USES: *C:* panacea or, as John Evelyn put it, 'a Catholicon against all infirmities';
  HER: eye baths, rheumatism, throat infections.

Elder or Elderberry was always associated with evil. Witches either had one growing in their gardens or they lived amongst its branches. This is one reason why it was rarely cut down and so the dank dark nutrient-enriched corners where it thrived got danker and darker. If an elder had to be trimmed, apologies had to be made first. The fruits are used in jams, jellies and preserves and for making wine, recommended to rejuvenate the elderly. The flowers are also used in wine-making and are components of eyewashes and also medicines for all sorts of bronchial complaints. The leaves, which contain alkaloids, were used as insecticides and compounded with linseed oil as a salve to reduce bruising.

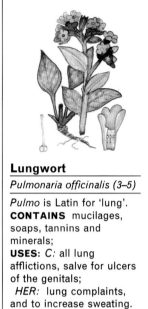

Vervain

(15) Verbena officinalis (6–9)

Valued by the Druids as second only to Mistletoe.
CONTAINS essential oils, bitters, mucilage and glycosides;
USES: *C:* magical cure-all;
  HER: wounds, diuretic, regularising periods and promoting the flow of milk; Bach.

Lungwort

Pulmonaria officinalis (3–5)

Pulmo is Latin for 'lung'.
CONTAINS mucilages, soaps, tannins and minerals;
USES: *C:* all lung afflictions, salve for ulcers of the genitals;
  HER: lung complaints, and to increase sweating.

Verbena is a corruption of the Latin *herba bona*, which means 'good plant' and the Vervain and others of its genus have been employed throughout history for all manner of good uses. The Romans looked to it as a good omen and the crusaders reckoned that it had sprung up from beneath the Cross. If it was to be collected for use, words of thanks had to be said and gifts of honey, still in the comb, given to the soil. To take a bath in Vervain allowed you to see into the future and so obtain all your desires, while its leaves pressed into a small cut in your hand allowed all doors to be opened.

The spotted leaves of Lungwort stand out along any roadside and, as they resemble a lung, the plant was used to treat all manner of complaints of the chest. The milk-white spots were attributed to the milk of the Virgin Mary and the flowers, which change from rose-pink through mauve to blue, add to the mystery of the plant.

Chamomile should really be called Roman Chamomile because it was probably introduced by them into Britain. It was used as a strewing herb to cover the floors and the malodours of medieval life. In Tudor times it became a fragrant favourite for the creation of lawns, ousting the grasses as a protective coverall, being equally tolerant of treading and clipping. One of the great lawns at Buckingham Palace which each year bears the brunt of thousands of feet at the most famous garden parties of all is made of this plant; although the tea served there is Earl Grey, itself flavoured with the essential oil of the Bergamot Orange.

Chamomile

(6) Anthemis nobilis (6–7)

CONTAINS an essential oil which includes chamazulene, coumarins, heterosides and esters of angelic acid; no wonder it makes you feel so good!
USES: *C:* prevents internal cramps, a digestive and rejuvenative;
  HER: migraine, neuralgia, calming the digestive system and cooling fevers.

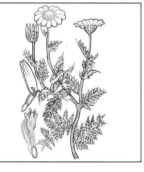

Chamomile is said to revive plants which are lucky enough to grow near it and as a ptisane it is a great reviver of people, as Gerard wrote, 'It is a special helpe against wearisomnesse, it easeth and mitigateth paine, it mollifieth and suppleth'. Today it is one of the favourite herbal teas on sale and is the main constituent of a number of herbal formulations, including a wash to brighten tired and broken hair.

Fortunately, the management of our roadside heritage has recently become more enlightened, and in places mowing takes place only after the flowers have had a chance to set seed. So today a drive along even a new motorway can be lined with floral and herbal fascination, but please, only for the passengers.

GRASSLANDS

Grasslands are probably our most ancient people-made and managed habitat, produced by increased grazing pressure long before the mechanical lawn-mower was invented. The floral diversity of the end product is not only due to the intensity of management but also to the nature of the underlying bedrock, with acid grasslands tending to be at one end of the spectrum and limestone and chalk grasslands at the other.

Acid grasslands are often floristically poor and are dominated by two inedible plants, Mat-grass and Sweet Vernal-grass. The former is so wiry and tough that it appears to be just not worth the effort, the latter is flavoured with trouble and the taste of new-mown hay. The

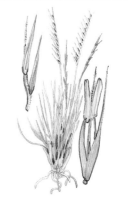

Mat-grass

Nardus stricta (6–8)

Avoided by animals, it is the main healer of our acidified, overgrazed uplands for it takes over and protects the soil from erosion. If you see its bleached, comb-like rhizomes and leaf-bases lying on the surface of the soil where they have been rooted up by desperate sheep, it is a sure sign of overgrazing and mismanagement. It is a plant whose medicinal virtues have not yet been discovered.

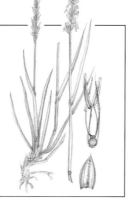

Sweet Vernal-grass

(Poison ×) Anthoxanthum odoratum (4–6)

A very common grass found on acid, neutral and limestone grassland, both wet and dry. Sowerby and Johnson in their book *Grasses of Great Britain* (1851–67) ask: 'Whether its wide distribution may not be productive of some wholesome medicinal effects on the more promiscuously feeding grazing animals'?
CONTAINS coumarins.

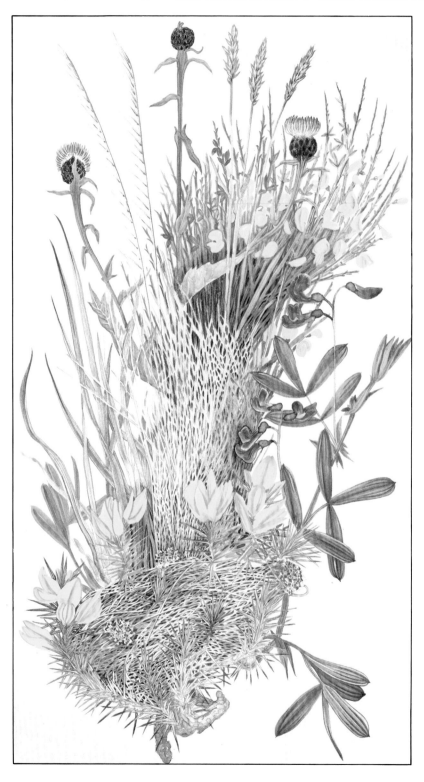

Acid Grassland – sweet and sour medicine

1 Gorse, *Ulex europaeus*
2 Hardheads, *Centaurea nigra*
3 Mat-grass, *Nardus stricta*
4 Sweet Vernal-grass, *Anthoxanthum odoratum*
5 Broom, *Sarothamnus scoparius*
6 Bitter Vetch, *Lathyrus montanus*
7 Dodder, *Cuscuta epithymum*

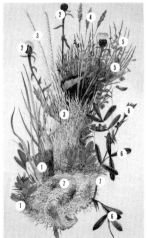

flavour is due to a chemical, coumarin, which comes in more than 100 different forms, producing a sickly-sweet fricassee which gives cattle the staggers if eaten in too large an amount.

Hardheads, a thistle-like member of the Daisy Flower Family, often dominates the scene in the early stages of acidification. Girls would collect one of the hardheads to use as a love oracle. First they would pull off any opened flowers, then they would place the plant in their bosom and think about the man they hoped loved them. After one hour, if a new flower had opened all would be well and love would come their way from the right quarter.

Thanks in part to acidification brought on by land mismanagement and acid rain, Tormentil is now one of our commonest plants. As we have already seen (page 64), it is prized in the Highlands and Islands of Scotland as a source of tannin for tanning. At the other end of Scotland in the borders, evidence is being unearthed at Soutra Hospital showing that the plant was used to rid people of intestinal worms. The proof is in the excavation, where remains of Tormentil and the cysts of the worms are found together in high concentration, real bedpan fellows.

Another plant prized in the Highlands was the Bitter Vetch. Their swollen underground

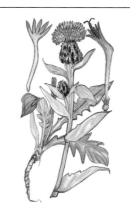

Hardheads

Centaurea nigra (6–9)

Cheiron the Centaur is said to have used the Knapweeds as a wound herb.
CONTAINS bitters and tannins;
USES: *C:* healing wounds, especially those of the nose and mouth;
HER: sore throats, catarrh, and for treating bruises and ruptures.

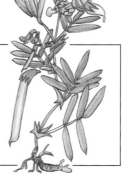

Bitter Vetch

Lathyrus montanus (4–7)

Eaten in many parts of Scotland under the names of Cormeille and Dio, the roots have a very similar taste to chestnuts when roasted. There is no record of its use in medicine, one can only wonder why.

parts were dug up to be eaten either cooked or raw and were also chewed to enhance the flavour of whisky. William Turner (1520–1568), the renowned English botanist, wrote,

The Nuts of this Pease being boiled and eaten, are hardlier digested then be either Turneps or Parsneps, yet do they nourish no lesse then the Parsneps: they are not so windie as they, they do more slowly passe thorowe the belly by reason of their binding qualitie, and being eaten rawe, they be yet harder of digestion, and do hardlier and slowlier descend.

Gorse and Broom are two more members of the same flower family. Many plants in this family have root nodules infested with nitrogen-fixing bacteria so they are often themselves rich in nitrogen, one reason why they grow so well even in acid places and contain many poisonous chemicals. Despite this, the family has given us the Peas and Beans on which we all depend for the protein-building part of our diet.

Gorse, though producing a riot of colour in late summer, provides the bees with a few flowers throughout the year and the herbalist with a cupboard full of remedies. Dry Gorse burns well and the Druids lit fires of it to celebrate the spring equinox; beacons in high places. In the same way, blazing Gorse branches were carried among cattle on Midsummer night to ward off future evil. Used as an armoured hedging plant, it protected cattle and sheep from attack by predators, but it is itself attacked by the strange parasitic plant called Dodder.

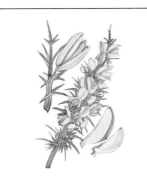

Gorse

Ulex europaeus (3–6)

Gorst in Old English signified a 'waste place' in which nothing of use would grow.
CONTAINS alkaloids and flavones.
USES: once valued in Ireland as fodder for working horses, kitchen fuel and for its ash; the bark and flowers produce a yellow dye (the yellow used in many Scottish tartans);
 C: Jaundice and kidney problems; Bach.

Dodder

Cuscuta epithymum (7–9)

'Kechout' is an Arabic word from which *Cuscuta* is derived.
CONTAINS anthracenosides which are taken up from the small intestine and react some six hours later by causing the large intestine to contract;
USES: *C:* a number of internal disorders especially those of the intestine, also as a contraceptive.

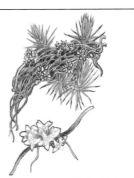

The winding stems of Dodder, in sharp contrast to the straight spikiness of Gorse from which it draws its nourishment, signalled intestines to Dioscorides, who prescribed it for constipation under the name of Epithumon. He believed that the virtues of Dodder changed with the host and so prescribed Dodder from Thyme for spleenful headaches and the itch, and Dodder from Nettles as a diuretic. Since that time these have been shown to be two separate species, not the same plant.

In heraldry, Broom signifies knighthood and it was the emblem of the Plantagenets down to the time of Richard III in the fifteenth century. In parts of France people pickle the flower-buds just as they open and use them as a good substitute for Capers; while in the Auvergne they believe that sheep who eat the plant become immunised against snakebites. There is some back-up evidence for the latter, as the plant has long been used as an antidote to a number of poisons.

Of course, it was also used for making brooms but never with the flowers on or death of the head of the house would ensue. It was a magical plant with aphrodisiacal properties and was used as a processional strewing herb at weddings and in church decoration. It was never collected during the merry month of May.

The Yorkshire sage and scholar Alcuin, 735–804, grew Broom beside his cell, where it was the home for an ill-fated nightingale. Alcuin is said to have taught the more famous Charlemagne much about herbal lore.

Lime has long been used as an antidote to acidity both by adding it to the land and by taking it internally for heartburn. Limestone and chalk help to provide great relief in the countryside for it is on outcrops of these rocks that we can find our most diverse and beautiful grassland.

Fairy Flax, despite its diminutive size, is a very powerful purge. In Ireland it is called *Lion na mban sidhe* or the Fairy Women's Flax, linking the wise women herbalists with strange things beyond the ken of the average mortal.

Violets, especially scented ones, are flowers of Venus and her son Priapus, the God of gardens and generation. Yet so famous was the Violet as an emblem of love and affection that many other deities laid claim to connections with the flowers. They were thought to have sprung from the blood of Ajax and of Attis; and were also the food of a daughter of Ianchus beloved of Jupiter who turned her into a heifer. In Celtic times, Violets were known by cuckoo names – Cuckoo's Shoe and Cuckoo's Stockings – again linking them to spring and sex.

Chicory is a salad or

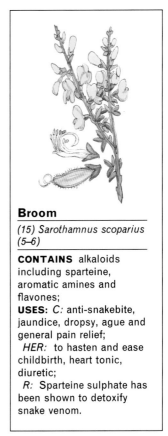

Broom

(15) *Sarothamnus scoparius* (5–6)

CONTAINS alkaloids including sparteine, aromatic amines and flavones;
USES: *C:* anti-snakebite, jaundice, dropsy, ague and general pain relief;
 HER: to hasten and ease childbirth, heart tonic, diuretic;
 R: Sparteine sulphate has been shown to detoxify snake venom.

Fairy Flax

Linum catharticum (6–9)

Catharticum means 'purging' and Gerard counselled that the violent action of this little plant should be diluted with white wine.
CONTAINS essential oils, bitters, tannin and a resin;
USES: *HER:* emetic (causing vomiting) and a blood purifier;
 HOM: bronchitis, to regularise periods, and for piles.

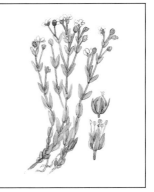

root vegetable and that's exactly what the Greek *kichore* means. The blue flower and the plant which bears it is in contrast to the forced White Whitloof and Endive forms, both of which add a certain bitterness to salads and to synthetic coffee. Another name is Succory,

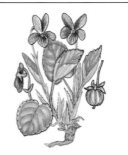

Chicory

Cichorium intybus (7–9)

A magical plant, grown as an aphrodisiac and pulled out of the ground with a stag's horn or a piece of gold. Collected in strict silence on 27 June or 25 July, the days of St Peter and St James.
CONTAINS a surfeit of the sugar inulin, a number of bitters and latex;
USES: salad and pot herb;
 C: aphrodisiac, eye tonic and diuretic;
 HER: dropsy, jaundice, stimulates the bile and for digestive cramps; Bach.

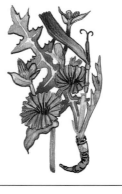

Sweet Violet

(7) Viola odorata (4–5)

Pliny believed that the colour of the flowers was a sure cure for headaches and migraine, while Gerard spoke more of their beauty 'bringing to men's minds ... the rememberance of honestie, comlinesse and all kinds of virtues'.
CONTAINS soaps, mucilages, odoratine (an alkaloid), blue pigments, and irone which provides the scent;
USES: *C:* epilepsy, pleurisy, quinsy, jaundice, and for inducing sleep;
 HER: respiratory disorders, to clear the bronchi and as a mild purgative.

the beautiful young girl who spurned the amorous intentions of the Sun and so was turned into a plant which had to stand and stare aloft throughout the hours of daylight. The flowers do open and close with the sun and water distilled from Chicory flowers was used to treat inflammation and dimness of the eyes. If laid upon an anthill the flowers are rapidly turned a brilliant red.

One of our loveliest limestone grassland plants is the Pasque Flower, always rare and getting rarer, and always associated with ancient earthworks and battles – again linked to Danish blood. The flower, though a wonderful paschal-blue, yields a bright green dye traditionally used to dye hens' eggs at Paschal-tide. The same species has been used for thousands of years in Chinese medicine to cure a variety of ills from malaria to madness.

Pasque Flower

(Poison ×××) Pulsatilla vulgaris (3–5)

One plant which should never have been called 'vulgar', for it has great elegance and beauty.
CONTAINS soaps, tannins and ranunculosides which become inactive on drying and heating.
USES: *HER:* sedative, diuretic, anti-cramps, to cause sweating, and as an external warming rub;
 HOM: tincture for many complaints from migraine, skin infections to poly-arthritis.

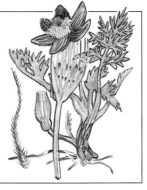

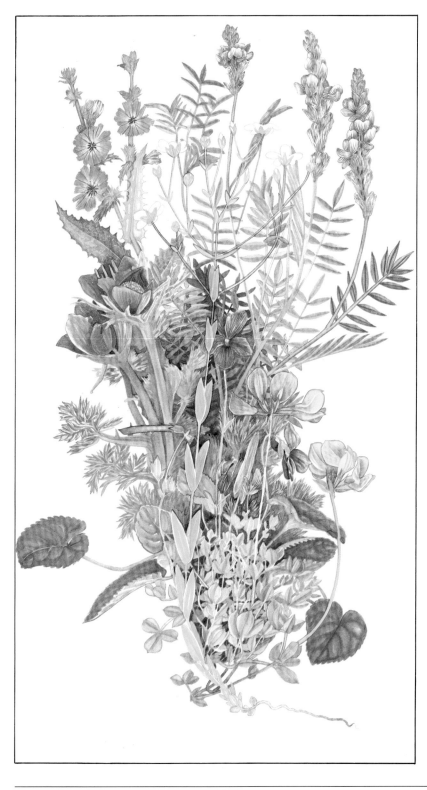

Lime Rich Grassland

1 Sweet Violet, *Viola odorata*
2 Fairy Flax, *Linum catharticum*
3 Pasque Flower, *Pulsatilla vulgaris*
4 Chicory, *Cichorium intybus*
5 Sainfoin, *Onobrychis viciifolia*
6 Bird's-foot Trefoil, *Lotus corniculatus*

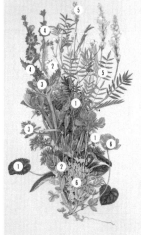

The strangely named Sainfoin is one of my favourite plants as it finds its northern limit not far from my home in County Durham. Like me, it is a displaced southerner for it gets commoner and more abundant on limestones the further you travel south, down into Europe. It is arguably our most beautiful native member of the Pea Flower Family with, as Geoffrey Grigson so aptly puts it, its flowers of Quattrocento Pink: the pink of the blooms which are said to have sprouted from the hay on which the Baby Jesus lay in the manger.

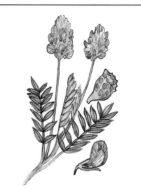

Sainfoin

Onobrychis viciifolia (6–8)

Sainfoin is French for 'Holy Hay'. Gerard spurned its use but Culpeper, perhaps confusing it with the *Onobruchus* of Dioscorides, used it to bring on a sweat, for cleaning boils and as a diuretic. He reckoned that, 'It is a singular food for Cattel causing them to give great store of milk, and why then may it not be the lyke being boyled in ordinary drink for nurses.'

Bird's-foot Trefoil

Lotus corniculatus (6–9)

When massed on a hillside its fragrance is sickly sweet. Despite its abundance and its many common names it appears to have been little used in medicine except as a binder against diarrhoea and for staunching the flow of blood.

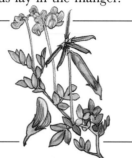

To complete this brief list of limestone healers we have another member of the Pea Flower Family, Bird's-foot Trefoil or take your pick from seventy other common names. Geoffrey Grigson asks why this very common plant should have so many names when others equally common, such as Tufted Vetch, have but a few. Though he finds no answer to his question, he jogs our memory back to those times when witchcraft was not a figment of television imagery but a real source of fear to people of town and especially the countryside. The black twisted claw-like fruits which replace the flowers of Bird's-foot Trefoil, though cradled in beauty, also hinted of strange powers in their seeds. Wise women who knew their herbs gave wise counsel in their use; but the claws of witchcraft sent so many kindly women, and the knowledge they had, to oblivion at the stake.

PASTURES AND MEADOWS

Grassland is traditionally any place where animals were grazed for part of the year: acid outbyeland, the unenclosed moorland beyond the stonewalls of the Pennines, or downland of the chalk and limestone in the south. Pasture consists, more often than not, of enclosed fields in which animals graze with contentment on flower-rich grassland;

while meadow, again traditionally enclosed, was kept to grow a crop of hay for winter feed. Meadows allowed all the plants to complete their cycle of reproduction – flowering, fruiting and setting seed – so ensuring a good diverse crop in the following year. The animals were then pastured on the regrowth before being fed on the hay, and so played their part by returning organic nutrients to the soil. Best and most diverse of all were the water-meadows which used to flank all our rivers and streams because they had the extra benefit of winter flooding, complete with a large input of mineral-rich silt, free fertiliser.

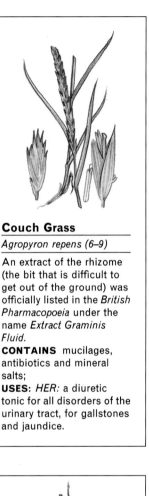

Couch Grass

Agropyron repens (6–9)

An extract of the rhizome (the bit that is difficult to get out of the ground) was officially listed in the *British Pharmacopoeia* under the name *Extract Graminis Fluid.*
CONTAINS mucilages, antibiotics and mineral salts;
USES: *HER:* a diuretic tonic for all disorders of the urinary tract, for gallstones and jaundice.

PASTURES

Couch Grass and Field Horsetail are both common in our pastures and, unfortunately, in our gardens where thanks to their deep spreading roots they are, as Anne Pratt says, 'most difficult of extirpation and will retain their vitality amid many injuries'. The word couch comes from an Anglo-Saxon word which means 'holding on to life'. The roots are full of a strange sweetness and ideal for brewing beer. This is good news, because before you had extirpated enough to do the job you would indeed have a great thirst. A water extract of the rhizome has been used since the Middle Ages to ease cystitis and other urinary problems and has recently come back into great favour.

Field Horsetail is another noxious garden weed. Like all the other members of the Horsetail clan, its nearest relatives are, or rather were, giant plants which lived millions of years ago and formed much of the coal and anthracite we use today. They were eminently fossilisable thanks to the high concentrations of silica found in their stems and leaves. Silicon is the second commonest element

Field Horsetail

Equisetum arvense (3–4)

Keeping your garden free from this noxious weed will certainly help to keep you fit, for it is hard physical labour.
CONTAINS silica, flavonoids, soaps and even a trace of that dreaded alkaloid nicotine;
USES: pan scrubbers and pot scourers in the days before Teflon-coated utensils;
 C: diuretic, kidney stones, and in the treatment of tuberculosis;
 HER: cystitis and pulmonary tuberculosis;
 R: good source of silica and other minerals which strengthen eyesight and the skeletal system.

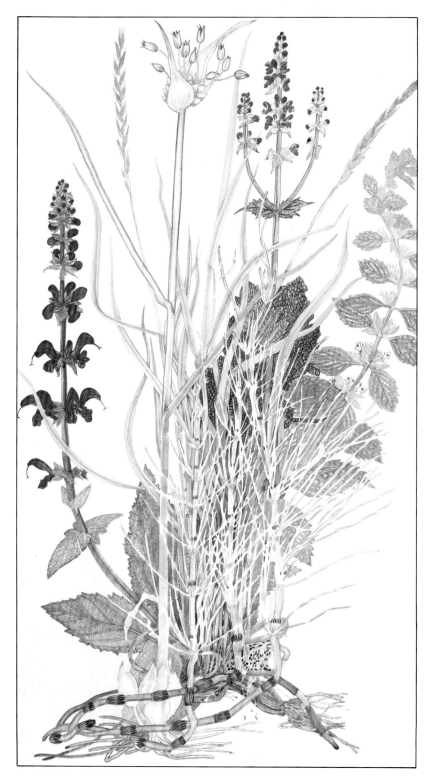

Pastures – in which the animals may safely graze

1 Field Horsetail, *Equisetum arvense*
2 Meadow Sage, *Salvia pratensis*
3 Couch Grass, *Agropyron repens*
4 Wild Onion, *Allium vineale*
5 Wild Clary, *Salvia horminoides*
6 Bee Balm, *Melissa officinalis*

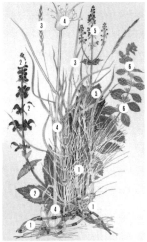

after oxygen on the face of the Earth. It is an important constituent of the clays which bind soils together and hold other essential elements making them available for uptake by growing plants. Recent research by Louis Kervran, a French biochemist, has shown that silica is very important in many aspects of the health of human beings and that our modern Horsetails are a good source of supply.

Four members of the Dead-nettle Family make up a bouquet fit to garnish the product of any pasture. Wild Clary, one of a number of plants whose seeds take on a frogspawn consistency when soaked in water, was used as organic eye drops; evidently with great success, for the plant came to be known as 'Christ's Eye'.

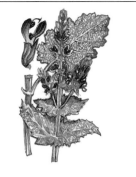

Wild Clary

(3) Salvia horminoides (6–9)

Salveo is Latin for 'I heal' and *clarus* means 'clear'. Clary has much the same content, action and uses as Sage. Clary seeds beaten into a powder and taken in wine were thought to be aphrodisiac.

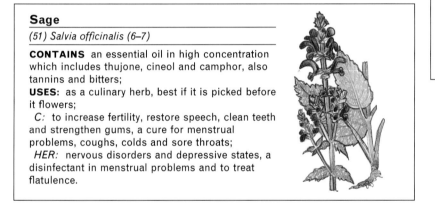

Sage

(51) Salvia officinalis (6–7)

CONTAINS an essential oil in high concentration which includes thujone, cineol and camphor, also tannins and bitters;
USES: as a culinary herb, best if it is picked before it flowers;
  C: to increase fertility, restore speech, clean teeth and strengthen gums, a cure for menstrual problems, coughs, colds and sore throats;
  HER: nervous disorders and depressive states, a disinfectant in menstrual problems and to treat flatulence.

Clary is a native plant but the larger and more pungent Sage was introduced, probably from France, very early on. It became one of the soothing mainstays of medieval medicine and was the most popular plant with the Physicians of Myddfai who included it in no fewer than fifty-two of their prescriptions by kind permission of the Lady of the Lake for it was said to thrive 'only where there was a domineering wife'. One strange property of Sage is its ability to stop perspiration for several days; it is also said to do the same for milk production and has oestrogenic properties.

Bee Balm, beloved of bees and herbalists alike, was planted near hives to keep the precious insects from straying too far from home. The flowering tips of the plant were steeped in white wine along with lemon rind, cinnamon, cloves, nutmeg and coriander to form the basis of Eau des Carmes, which was the original Eau de Cologne, made by the Carmelite monks in the seventeenth century. Culpeper wrote that 'It causeth the heart to become merry', and Llewellyn, Prince of Glamorgan, is said to have lived to the ripe old age of 108, thanks to this plant.

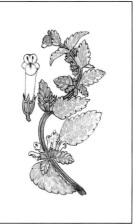

Bee Balm

(2) Melissa officinalis (6–8)

Melisophyllon is the Greek for 'beloved by bees'.
CONTAINS an essential oil which includes linalol, geraniol and citrol;
USES: lemon flavouring for food, and lemon scent for furniture polish;
 C: for any complaints including heaviness of the heart, also to calm the spirit and the stomach;
 HER: a stimulant, a perspirant, anti-cramps and a sedative. Modern herbal teas made from this plant reputedly relieve headaches, lift tiredness, and calm the nervous system while stimulating the heart.

Marjoram completes this 'coven' of kitchen herbs and witches were said to use it as a cleansing bath each spring. Its flowers produce a dye which turns purple on wool and brown on linen; and the herb was tied in sprigs to milk churns to stop the milk going sour in thundery weather.

No kitchen garden would be complete without the Onion and its kin. It has been used as a food and as a disinfectant and bacteriostat, both internal and external, since the dawn of cooking and medicine. During the First World War people were asked to grow Garlic on a massive scale for use as a wound disinfectant in the trenches; all part of the home front war effort. The gardeners of Britain responded well and, at a King's shilling a pound, some made good money until the market was flooded.

Two women of the time were at the forefront of the war effort both for their country and for their calling, herbal medicine. They were Mary Grieve and Hilda Leyel, and in a large garden in Buckinghamshire they grew Garlic among more than 300 other healing herbs. Before the war, supplies of healing plants had traditionally come from the Continent and so once war broke out the situation was desperate. The ladies and their pupils responded magnificently.

In the post-war years, continued interest in the herbal aspects of medicine led to the founding in 1927 of the Society of Herbalists, with its headquarters where else but at Culpeper House in Bruton Street,

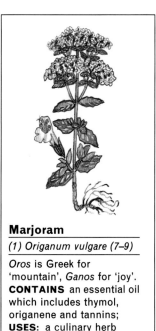

Marjoram

(1) Origanum vulgare (7–9)

Oros is Greek for 'mountain', *Ganos* for 'joy'.
CONTAINS an essential oil which includes thymol, origanene and tannins;
USES: a culinary herb especially with fish dishes;
 C: snuff to clear the head, used with honey to remove bruises and skin blemishes, as a warming rub for stiff joints;
 HER: whooping and other violent coughs, and in relaxing herbal baths.

London W1. The 1930s were, however, to see the new wonderdrugs, synthetics and antibiotics, oust herbs, herbals and herbalism into a backwater of popular concern. I am sure that the two formidable ladies would be glad to have seen the revival of so many of their ideas and beliefs seventy years on, and would welcome and applaud the new research on Garlic which is showing that the virtues are still in place.

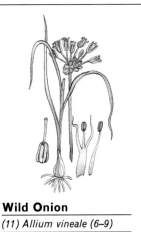

MEADOWS

One man went to mow,
Went to mow a meadow,

but only after the flowers had all set seed. Today, unfortunately, most of our ancient pasture and meadows have been ploughed and re-seeded with Perennial Rye-grass, which is cropped for hay and silage.

Wild Onion

(11) Allium vineale (6–9)

There are a number of Wild Onion species from which the whole range of garden varieties is derived, including Chives, Leeks and Garlic.
CONTAINS sulphur heterosides, the tear-jerking aroma is in part due to allyl-propyl disulphide, also flavones, enzymes and vitamins A, B and C;
USES: as a vegetable and as flavouring, and as a general antiseptic and pick-you-up.
  R: underway.

Darnel

(Poison ××) Lolium temulentum (6–9)

CONTAINS temuline in its ripe seeds, an alkaloid which induces sleep and vertigo. It also paralyses the nerve centres which regulate the action of the lungs and so causes acute breathing difficulties;
USES: *HOM:* rheumatism, arthritis, neuralgia, internal cramps, sickness and trembling limbs.

Darnel, a close relative of Rye-grass, has the strange distinction of being our only poisonous grass. Opinion varies on this point from the ancient laws of China which ban its use in brewing to superstitions which say it becomes a problem only when used for fermentation or when bread made with it is eaten while still hot. Modern research has shown that it does contain alkaloids which induce sleep and giddiness. The now rampant Perennial Rye contains several alkaloids, perhaps even more now under today's intensive cultivation which requires the massive use of nitrogen.

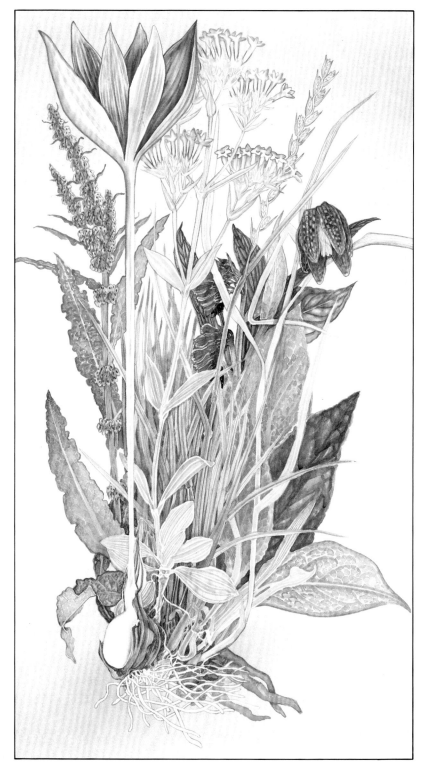

Pastures Old – producing a sweet diversity of hay

1 Meadow Saffron, *Colchicum autumnale*
2 Dock, *Rumex crispus*
3 Common Centaury, *Centaurium erythrea*
4 Darnel, *Lolium temulentum*
5 Comfrey, *Symphytum officinale*
6 Fritillary, *Fritillaria meleagris*

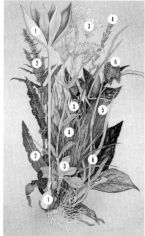

The recorded use of Comfrey goes back more than 2000 years when it was first named by Dioscorides as *Symphytum*, as in symphony, which means 'to join together in harmony'. The plant was used as a salve to help reduce bruising and to mend broken bones.

Gerard advises us, 'The slimie substance of the

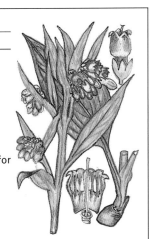

Comfrey

(2) (Poison ××) Symphytum officinale (5–7)

CONTAINS a number of alkaloids including symphyto-cynoglossine, pyrrolizidine, tannins, starch and the sugar asparagine;
USES: as an organic fodder plant;
 C: as a poultice to heal bones, certainly if enough was applied it could act like a soft plaster of Paris;
 HER: as a poultice for a range of complaints, pleurisy, bronchitis and rheumatism, as a cream for cuts, burns and varicose veins, a gargle for sore throats and as an enema and douche to relieve soreness and pain;
 R: provides evidence that it promotes the reduction of bruising and healing.

roote made in a posset of ale, and given to drinke against the paine in the backe, gotten by any violent motion, as wrestling and over much use of women, doth in fower or five daies perfectly cure the same, although the involuntarie flowing of the seed in men be gotten thereby.' A plant with a sting in its tale, and so it has: once grown extensively as animal fodder and recommended as an organic cleansing mulch, its internal use in tablets and capsules has now been banned. It is genetically very diverse (hence its names such as Abraham, Isaac and Jacob, referring to its varied flower colour) and certain varieties contain poisons. We should again heed the warning that herbal medicine is safe only in the hands of the trained practitioner and we should recognise that continued research is required to clear the name even of the oldest remedy. It must also be borne in mind that the massive applications of nitrogen used in intensive agriculture today may well put even our common plants under stress, changing their own internal biochemistry, for better or for worse.

Nitrate in itself is not a poison but too much, once in the food chain, can cause havoc. During the digestive process in ruminants, and unfortunately also in human infants, bacteria which normally aid the process of digestion can turn nitrate into nitrite. Nitrite is a poison for it suppresses the oxygen-carrying capacity of the red haemoglobin in our blood turning it, and the baby, blue. This is one reason why the World Health Authority does its best to set stringent limits on the amount of nitrogen in drinking water.

The destruction of ancient grassland swards by ploughing released an enormous quantity of nitrogen, normally held fast in the natural cycle, down on its way to the ground water. This effect, magnified by continued use of more and more fertiliser to boost the crops and the fact that we no longer burn the stubble in the fields but allow it to rot *in situ* thus feeding the nitrogen-fixing bacteria, all bode more trouble in the future both for the plants and for us.

Meadow Saffron, Autumn Crocus or Naked Lady, so-called because its flower is unprotected by any leaves as it erupts from a corm which may be twenty-five centimetres below the soil, is not the Saffron used as a culinary colourant and is not the common Crocus which belongs to an entirely different plant family. Meadow Saffron is a member of the Lily Flower Family and it contains a deadly poison, colchicine, which arrests cell division and kills by 'strangulation', hence another of its names is plant arsenic. Yet used with care, it was shown to have many virtues, for in the past it was used as a painkiller and to treat gout.

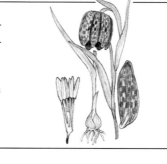

Meadow Saffron

(6) (Poison ××××)
Colchicum autumnale (8–9)

Colchis in classical mythology was a place famed for its medicinal plants.
CONTAINS the alkaloid colchicine, which stops the multiplication of living cells, also mucilages;
USES: *C|HER:* acute arthritis, gout and rheumatism, and used in the form of syrups for lung complaints.

Fritillary

(Poison ××××) Fritillaria meleagris (4–5)

Meleagris is the Latin word for 'guinea fowl' and both the bloom and the bird share the same speckled look.
CONTAINS the alkaloid imperialine which is extremely poisonous. To date not used in medicine; apart from its strange beauty its virtues await discovery.

Another poisonous member of the same family is the Snake's-head Fritillary which, like Meadow Saffron, was much commoner in the past, being especially abundant in the water-meadows of the Thames Valley. Argument goes on to this day regarding its status as a native plant because this striking flower was only first recorded in the late seventeenth century in a meadow not far from what is now Heathrow Airport.

Centaury, called *Keym Chreest* on the Isle of Man, is a blessed herb in the Celtic west for it was said to have grown in the footsteps of Christ on his way to Calvary. Full of bitter virtues, like so many other members of the Gentian Flower Family, it cleansed the body of many bitter things and healed wounds into the bargain. Its healing properties were first used by the legendary Cheiron the Centaur, which is where it derived its Latin name, *Centaurium*.

In the thirteenth century the German scholar Albertus Magnus recorded the following strange fact: 'Magicians assure us that this herb has a singular virtue for if it is mixed with the flood of a female hoopoe [a bird which rarely visits Britain] and put in a lamp with the oil, all those present will see themselves upside-down with their feet in the air.' Despite such ridiculous assertions the plant remained a mainstay of herbal medicine for many centuries.

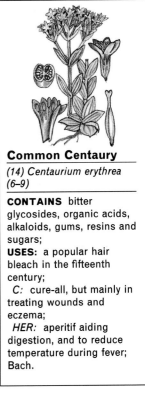

Common Centaury

(14) Centaurium erythrea (6–9)

CONTAINS bitter glycosides, organic acids, alkaloids, gums, resins and sugars;
USES: a popular hair bleach in the fifteenth century;
  C: cure-all, but mainly in treating wounds and eczema;
  HER: aperitif aiding digestion, and to reduce temperature during fever;
Bach.

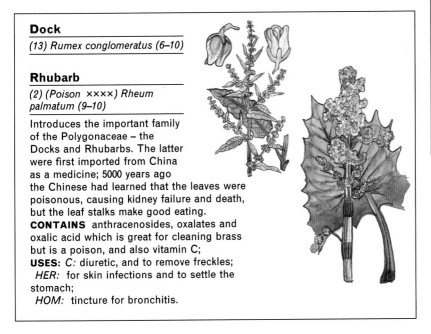

Dock

(13) Rumex conglomeratus (6–10)

Rhubarb

(2) (Poison ××××) Rheum palmatum (9–10)

Introduces the important family of the Polygonaceae – the Docks and Rhubarbs. The latter were first imported from China as a medicine; 5000 years ago the Chinese had learned that the leaves were poisonous, causing kidney failure and death, but the leaf stalks make good eating.
CONTAINS anthracenosides, oxalates and oxalic acid which is great for cleaning brass but is a poison, and also vitamin C;
USES: *C:* diuretic, and to remove freckles;
  HER: for skin infections and to settle the stomach;
  HOM: tincture for bronchitis.

'Stung by a Nettle, reach for the Dock', so goes the old lore and certainly the juice of the latter will soothe the hurt of the former. In Chaucer's time the following rhyme had to be said if the cure was to be effective:

Nettle out, Dock in,
Dock remove the Nettle sting.

Try it yourself while applying the Dock leaf and you will find it takes about that time to work. Some lucky people are unaffected by Nettle stings, feeling no pain and showing no allergic reaction but for most of us the Dock gives blessed relief.

Docks themselves are often affected by fungal and viral diseases which spot and blotch the leaves with livid purple and brown marks making them look not unlike diseased lungs. This is why they were used in the past to relieve tuberculosis, pneumonia and other respiratory complains. They were also used as salves to clear acne and freckles.

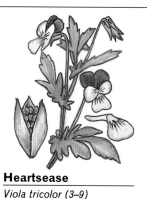

Heartsease

Viola tricolor (3–9)

It is called Heartsease because it was used in a cordial to help all conditions of the heart.
CONTAINS soaps, salicylates, flavones, pigments and coumarins;
USES: *C:* skin complaints and venereal diseases;
 HER: diarrhoea and urinary infections, skin problems especially in children.

FALLOW FIELDS

Fallow was a word which found its way into the English language when the arable fields were kept in good heart by wise crop rotation which included a period of rest. Even in my young days, fallow fields were a riot of colour and medicinal interest: yielding a bouquet of healing herbs which should perhaps begin with Heartsease and end with Ergot. Heartsease, which goes under many names including Meet-her-in-the-entry-kiss-her-in-the-buttery, was the plant whose juice Oberon squeezed into Titania's eyes, inducing her to fall in love with Bottom, the ass-headed weaver in Shakespeare's *Midsummer Night's Dream*.

Cupid is said to have shot an arrow into the flower which was originally white, giving it its three variable colours.

Poppy

(6) (Poison ×××) Papaver rhoeas (6–9)

All good members of the Poppy Flower Family produce coloured latex.
CONTAINS four aptly named alkaloids all with the prefix 'rhoe', mucilages and pigments;
USES: *C:* sedative and against migraine;
 HER: sedatives and to help coughs and colds.

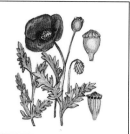

The real cupids were the gardeners who over the centuries reached into the hidden secrets of the Wild Pansies to give us the great range of velvet-flowered cultivars we have today. The herbalists were also not slow to latch on to the virtues of this shy beauty of the fallow fields which is also called Love-in-idleness. It was used for many purposes from cleansing the skin and easing the heart to treating venereal diseases.

The origin of the word Poppy is in some doubt: some say it comes

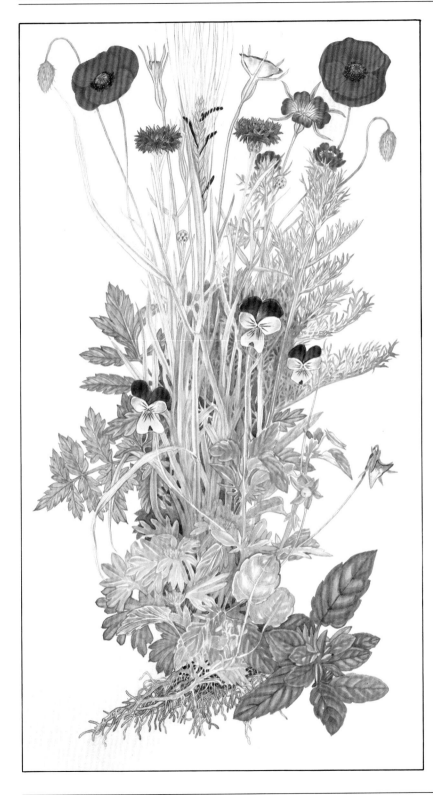

Flowers of Fallow Fields

1 Poppy, *Papaver rhoeas*
2 Rye (with Ergot), *Secale cereale*
3 Cornflower, *Centaurea cyanus*
4 Corn Cockle, *Agrostemma githago*
5 Pheasant's Eye, *Adonis annua*
6 Heartsease, *Viola tricolor*
7 Parsley Piert, *Aphanes arvensis*

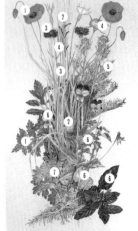

from the word *Papaver*, the Latin word for the plant; others that it comes from the Celtic *papa*, meaning pap or porridge, because the sap of the plant was mixed with gruel to hasten sleep in babies. The plant does not contain morphine but has always been used as a mild sedative. The Romans believed that Ceres, the Goddess of the harvest, was neglecting her duties to the detriment of food supplies. Somnus, God of sleep, came to the rescue by creating the somniferous Poppies which allowed Ceres to get enough sleep and so perform all her duties once again. No wonder the resting fallow fields are red with Poppies.

Introduced from Europe, the lovely Pheasant's Eye had joined the family of fallow field flowers by the fifteenth century. Gerard grew it in his London gardens as an ornamental under the name of Rose-a-Ruby. Later, it was sold by the street vendors crying 'Red Maracco'. It is a member of the Buttercup Flower Family and so was always collected early in the morning and used as quickly as possible for the best results. Thanks to the work of the Game Conservancy, wise land management practices which include leaving field edges, headlands and copses uncut and unsprayed make both the pheasant and the Pheasant's Eye more welcome in our countryside. Like the Foxglove, this plant was used to combat dropsy but it must be used with great care as it can kill by overstimulating the beating of the heart.

As the diminutive Parsley Piert, a member of the Rose Flower Family, grows on very stony ground it was highly regarded by the herb women around Bristol as a 'breakstone' for clearing the urinary tract. In Colonsay, off the west coast of Scotland, it was eaten pickled or raw as a salad, while in parts of England it was used to reduce inflammation of the bowels, or bowel hive, and colic in children.

The true Parsley is a very slow-growing member of the Carrot Flower Family, and it takes its name from *petros*, the Greek word for rock. It was one of the best known culinary herbs of early time. When you see it on your plate, don't just push it away but savour its virtues and its long history of use.

Pheasant's Eye

(Poison ××××) Adonis annua (4–5)

Its common name comes from the appearance of the flower.
CONTAINS several heart stimulants related to digitalin, and coumarin derivatives;
USES: *C/HER:* diuretic, sedative and heart tonic;
R: in 1963 it was found that all the heart-stimulating cardelonides appear to work by starving the heart of potassium. *Herba adonidis* works by causing the coronary blood vessels of the heart to dilate; used only for certain heart conditions.

Parsley Piert

Aphanes arvensis (4–10)

Also called Field Lady's Mantle. Although eaten as a salad and vegetable, it was not used in medicine; perhaps overlooked because of the introduction of the larger, more easily grown Parsley.
CONTAINS tannins, sugars and minerals.

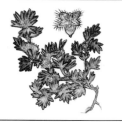

It is served as a side dish at the Jewish Feast of the Passover; and was also used for wreaths to crown the victors of the Isthmian Games in Greece, where it was also used to cover the dead and decorate graves. Shrouded in mystery, all sorts of superstitions revolved around the planting and plucking of Parsley, and yet it was widely used in medicine: eye-drops, eardrops, an aphrodisiac, against baldness and to dispel lumps which came with suckling a baby.

Josephine Addison records two ancient sayings in her *Illustrated Plantlore*, published in 1985, 'Only the wicked can grow Parsley' and 'Parsley only flourishes where Missus is Master'. Take your pick, but never give the plant away for your luck will go with it.

At the other end of the fallow field dispensary is the much-dreaded Ergot. If Rye infected with this parasite was baked into bread the results were horrific. The victims felt as if they were on fire, being pursued by wild beasts or even seeing flowers sprouting from their bodies. Hallucinogenic experiences, yes, but they were rapidly followed by miscarriage in pregnant women, gangrene of the legs, insanity and death. As recently as 1951 many people in a village in France died of ergotism, and many more recent reports are coming out from behind the now defunct Iron Curtain: it is a crop which must always be watched with care.

Parsley

(19) Petroselinum crispum (6–8)

Introduced from Europe as a year-round condiment and curative.
CONTAINS essential oils, flavones, vitamin C and protovitamin A;
USES: *C/HER:* baldness, menstrual problems, asthma, coughs, jaundice and dropsy, conjunctivitis and other eye complaints.

Ergot of Rye

(Poison ××××) Claviceps purpurea (7–8)

The black ergots are the resting stages of a parasitic fungus which takes over the ovary of the flower of cereals and other grasses. Under natural conditions they fall to the ground where they overwinter. The following spring each one produces thousands of spores which blow about on the wind, infecting other plants. Should the ergots be harvested with the grain the trouble begins. The Order of St Anthony was founded to care for affected people, who were thought to be not ill but possessed of demons.
CONTAINS a number of alkaloids including ergometrine which causes catastrophic contraction of the uterus.

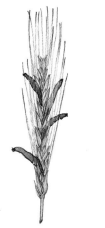

CHAPTER SIX

Plant hunting in the London scene

By the end of this sad century there will be more than six billion people trying to make a living off Planet Earth and more than 60 per cent of them will be living in an urban environment, divorced from any real contact with the healing powers of natural vegetation.

MARYLEBONE ROAD AND REGENT STREET

I was born off the Marylebone Road, London NW1 of mixed stock from Hoxton, Bethnal Green and Lambeth, and so it was to these places that I first returned to seek out the healing herbs of the urban scene.

The first I found was Coltsfoot, erupting through the tarmacadam at the base of a lamp-post, oblivious to the passing feet, belching traffic and piddling dogs. Its flowering spikes were past their prime and the new leaves, each one shaped like a tiny hoof, were well on their way, hence one of its other common names, Father-before-Son. Another name is Old Man's Baccy, for Pliny prescribed the smoke of the whole plant burned over Cypress charcoal and inhaled through a reed, with intermittent sipping of wine, as a remedy for the cough. Coltsfoot rock was prescribed for whooping-cough even in my young days, as was a trip to the local gas-works to inhale those coaltar vapours full of fossil anthracenes.

On the corner of Baker Street, thanks to an enterprising property developer who had flanked his refurbished mid high-rise with a truly wild garden, three more of the plants I sought were easy to come by.

The ever-so-common Chickweed tends to take over any free space.

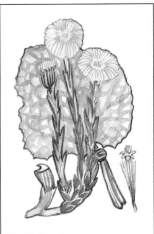

Coltsfoot

(3) Tussilago farfara (2–4)

Tussis comes from the Latin word for 'cough'.
CONTAINS mucilages and some sugars, inulin, galactose and pentose;
USES: from Classical times for coughs and respiratory complaints;
 HER: ptisanes against bronchitis, inflammation of the trachea, and chills.

My advice is to give it a chance and reap the benefit of year-round fresh mineral-rich salad, or cook it as a tasty substitute for Spinach. You could also overfeed it to your free-range hens and the whites of their eggs will turn an organic shade of green.

Yarrow is another of those common weeds, yet it is a plant so full of virtues that it really should be called by its proper name, *Achillea*. Achilles, so it is said, en route for Troy, wounded Telephus with his spear: a debilitating wound which was instantly cured by this plant which sprang up from the rust that fell from the offending weapon. *Achillea* has been used ever since as a wound herb to stem bleeding, both external and internal. One of its favourite haunts is the untidy corners of churchyards where it grows to rebuke the dead for not eating up their 'Yarrow broth'. It is a worthy plant indeed and across the centuries has been used as a love oracle in many different ways. Cut the stem and see for yourself, for there the initials of your loved one will be revealed for all with imagination to see.

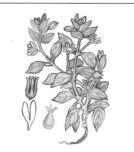

Chickweed

Stellaria media (1–12)

The name *stellaria* comes from its star-like flowers, some of the first and the last of each year.
CONTAINS soaps and minerals;
USES: *C:* boils and carbuncles, cramp, eye lotion, distilled and used as an aid to slimming with orange and lemon peel added;
 HER: external rub for rheumatic pains;
 HOM: rheumatism and psoriasis.

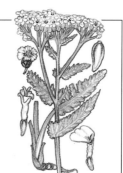

Yarrow

Achillea millefolium (5–10)

The young shoots give salad a tarragon-like tang.
CONTAINS an essential oil compounded with bitter achilleine, proazuline which helps cramps, and an antiseptic cineol. Together these give the plant its characteristic odour;
USES: bitters for brewing, seeds to preserve wine;
 C: to treat wounds;
 HER: tonic, for dyspepsia and anorexia.

Another name for Aaron's Rod is Mullein, possibly derived from the old English word *murrain*. It was used to treat a wide range of diseases in cattle and sheep. An infusion of its white-felted leaves was used as an antidote for animal diseases, especially of the lungs, which is where it got another name, Bullocky Lungwort. Under the name Clown's Lungwort it was used to treat the diseases which the 'ignorant' peasantry were supposed to have caught from the animals. One disease shared by man and beast, peasant and prince, was anthrax, now almost a terrible shadow of the past, thanks to the work of Louis Pasteur. He showed that many contagious diseases were caused by tiny bacteria which could be passed from one patient to another. In

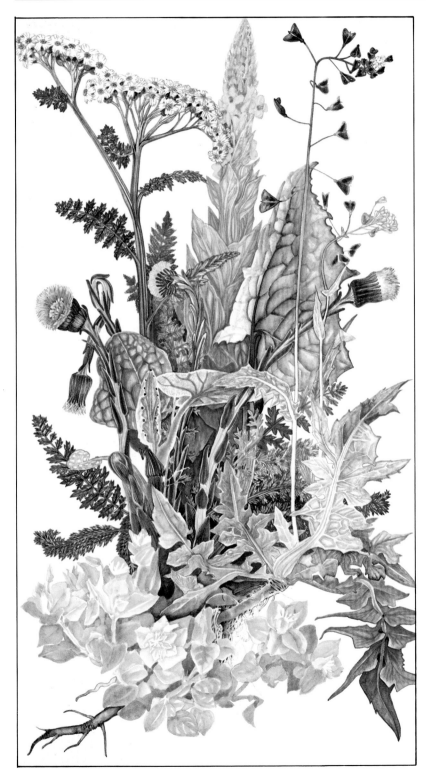

From Marylebone to Liverpool Street

1 Chickweed, *Stellaria media*
2 Yarrow, *Achillea millefolium*
3 Coltsfoot, *Tussilago farfara*
4 Aaron's Rod, *Verbascum thapsus*
5 Shepherd's Purse, *Capsella bursa-pastoris*

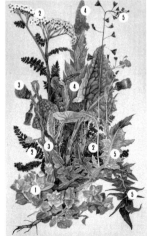

earlier times it had been common practice to slaughter diseased animals for human consumption, often with epidemic results; shades of today's mad cow disease.

SOHO

One name which should be remembered alongside that of Pasteur is John Snow, a London doctor whose detective work in Soho led him to the conclusion that cholera was contracted by drinking water polluted by human waste. He proved his point by removing the handle from what he knew to be the offending pump in Broadwick Street, so bringing London's last major cholera epidemic to an abrupt end. Paris celebrates the work of Pasteur with a great institute of learning and research, London remembers John Snow with a pub!

LIVERPOOL STREET STATION

Two hundred and thirty-eight years before the Broadwick Street revelation, Nicholas Culpeper was born in Surrey, the son of a vicar. He did well at school, excelled at Cambridge and seemed all set for a career either in the Church or in mainstream medicine. Fate would have it that he fell in love and decided to elope but his wife to be was killed on the way to their wedding, struck by lightning. Lovelorn and in disgrace, young Nicholas was apprenticed in the more lowly calling of apothecary. He eventually opened up his own shop in Spitalfields, previously home of high society but by then crumbling into a slum, and so set about a life's work of tending the local poor and pouring scorn on the mainstream medics and trendy apothecaries of his time. Well-read at Cambridge and well-versed in Latin, he saw through the sham of the establishment's so-called treatments which centred on very expensive concoctions often containing healing plants imported from abroad. He even had the audacity to translate their London Pharmacopoeia into good plain English, so blowing all their mumbo-jumbo Latin secrets.

Despite much acrimony and derision, on which he seemed to thrive, Culpeper finally published a do-it-yourself book of cures called *The English Physician*. Recommending the use of easily available local herbs,

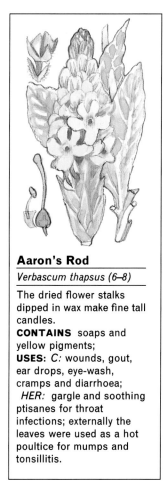

Aaron's Rod

Verbascum thapsus (6–8)

The dried flower stalks dipped in wax make fine tall candles.
CONTAINS soaps and yellow pigments;
USES: *C:* wounds, gout, ear drops, eye-wash, cramps and diarrhoea;
 HER: gargle and soothing ptisanes for throat infections; externally the leaves were used as a hot poultice for mumps and tonsillitis.

it was a great success and ran to no fewer than forty-seven editions, and is reprinted in facsimile form to this day.

Though Nicholas Culpeper was finally laid to rest in a churchyard upon which was built platform 11 of Liverpool Street Station, his work lives on: an inspiration to all the well-versed and well-trained herbalists who have been, and still are, called 'quacks' by some.

My diligent search of the newly-refurbished station concourse yielded nothing but plastic flowers made from non-renewable resources; yet given a chance and a smidgen of crumbling decay the wild plants will be back in force. There to prove it, not an olympic stone's throw from Culpeper's resting place, I found a tiny specimen of Shepherd's Purse, a fitting plant as it is also known as the Poor Man's Pharmacie. Of all our common plants this is one of the most variable, attaining full maturity complete with flowers and purse-shaped fruits in heights from just one to over fifty centimetres. If it was bound around the feet it was thought to cure jaundice; if used as drops of juice, to still the ringing in the ears; and applied in any form to stem bleeding from anywhere.

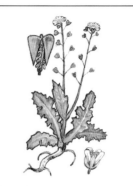

Shepherd's Purse

(3) Capsella bursa-pastoris (1–12)

With us around the year but its virtues fade if stored for more than twelve months. **CONTAINS** amino-alcohols and a flavonoid; **USES:** *C:* stops internal and external bleeding, sedative and jaundice; *HER:* earache, tinnitus and to treat wounds; *HOM:* for internal bleeding, cystitis and bladder complaints; *R:* the flavone diosmin backs up the action of the sympathetic nervous system and reduces blood pressure.

THE STRAND AND HIGH HOLBORN

John Gerard was born in Nantwich in 1545 and though he didn't get to Cambridge he made it into mainstream medicine, for at the age of fifty he was elected into the Court of the Barber Surgeon's Company. He was, above all, a great gardener and herbalist who knew his plants and prospered from their many virtues. His services were in great demand and he either ran, planned or owned gardens in the Strand, Holborn, Fetter Lane and on the east side of Mansion House. I searched in vain for plants in these places and recalled that, back in Gerard's time, London was no more than a series of villages interspersed with countryside; so he was able to collect Bugloss in Piccadilly, Clary in the fields of Holborn and Mallow hard by Tyburn. Never daunted, by searching the backstreets and especially the stairwells down to the basement flats below ground, once servants' quarters, it was not difficult to discover Ribwort Plantain, Elder, Groundsel, Daisy and Dandelion.

Turning to Gerard's *Herbal* published in 1597 we find this report of Ribwort Plantain,

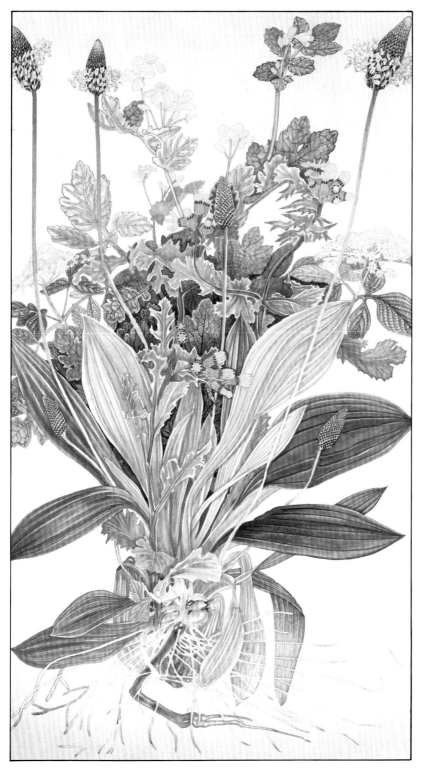

From the Strand to High Holborn

1 Groundsel, *Senecio vulgaris*
2 Ribwort Plantain, *Plantago lanceolata*
3 Greater Celandine, *Cheledonium majus*
4 Elder, *Sambucus nigra*

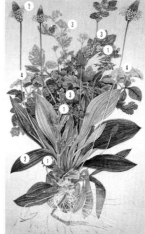

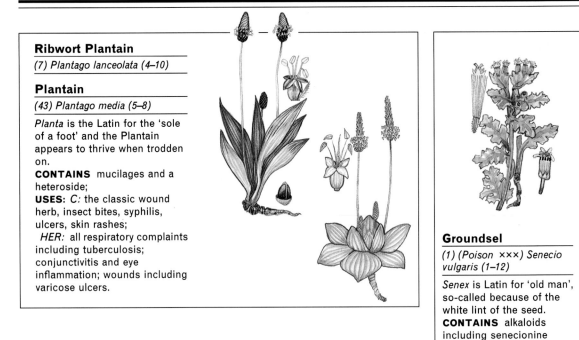

Ribwort Plantain

(7) Plantago lanceolata (4–10)

Plantain

(43) Plantago media (5–8)

Planta is the Latin for the 'sole of a foot' and the Plantain appears to thrive when trodden on.
CONTAINS mucilages and a heteroside;
USES: *C:* the classic wound herb, insect bites, syphilis, ulcers, skin rashes;
  HER: all respiratory complaints including tuberculosis; conjunctivitis and eye inflammation; wounds including varicose ulcers.

Groundsel

(1) (Poison ×××) Senecio vulgaris (1–12)

Senex is Latin for 'old man', so-called because of the white lint of the seed.
CONTAINS alkaloids including senecionine which damages the liver;
USES: *C:* sore throats, quinsy, catarrh and as a poultice for sciatica;
  HER: menstrual problems, nose bleeds;
  HOM: bladder infections.

The Juice dropped in the eies cooles the heate and inflammation thereof. I find in antient writers many good-morrowes, which I thinke not meet to bring into your memorie againe as That three roots will cure one griefe, four another disease – quarten ague – , six hanged about the necke are good for another maladye etc., all of which are but ridiculous toyes.

Well they may be, but even so I found this year in Wales the plant still in use as a wound dressing and for soothing varicose veins. Also Elder used to make a tonic wine from the flowers, and a cure for shingles made from the bark. Though Gerard may have scorned the stories of witches and evil long associated with this tree, he didn't turn his back on the medicine chest of the countryside and town, nor on the Groundsel plant which I found in abundance growing nearby.

The leaves of Groundsel boiled in wine or water and drunke, heal the paine and the ach of the stomacke that proceeds of Choler. Dioscorides saithe, That with the fine pouder of Frankincense, it healethe woundes in the sinues. The like operation hath the downe of the flowers mixed with vinegar.

Of 'Little Daiseys' Gerard has much to say, one set of virtues being as follows. 'The juice of the roots and leaves snift up the nosthrils purgeth the head mightily and helpeth the megrim. The

Daisy

(11) Bellis perennis (1–5)

CONTAINS soaps, mucilages, essential oil, tannins and bitters;
USES: *C:* to treat wounds, especially wounds of the breast and swelling of the testicles;
HER: expectorant, skin problems, jaundice;
HOM: skin and liver complaints.

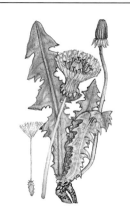

same given to little dogs with milke keepeth them from growing greate.' Perhaps yes to the former but rubbish to the latter, you might be tempted to say, as this little plant whose leaves we eat in salads and whose flowers we link in chains has a darker side to its nature.

Dwarfs and other oddities were in great demand in the courts of Renaissance times. As there were evidently not enough of the natural genetic variety to fill the bill as servants and entertainment, infants were abducted and fed on special milk-based diets laced with dwarfing herbs such as Daisy and Knotgrass. Did Shakespeare have prior knowledge of the information contained in Liceto's *De Monstrorum Causis*, or the causation of monsters, published in Italy in 1614, when he wrote:

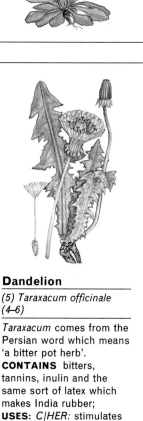

Dandelion

(5) Taraxacum officinale (4–6)

Taraxacum comes from the Persian word which means 'a bitter pot herb'.
CONTAINS bitters, tannins, inulin and the same sort of latex which makes India rubber;
USES: *C/HER:* stimulates the flow of bile and so helps treat cirrhosis of the liver. A great diuretic and so effective in dropsy, gallstones and as a general purifier of the body.

> Get you gone, you dwarf,
> You minimus of hindering knot-grass made,

or was the practice of dwarfing children one of those post-medieval nastinesses that was only hinted at in the polite society which both Gerard and Shakespeare served?

Current research shows this to be no ghoulish fairy-tale as all the dwarfing plants listed in the medieval manuscripts have been shown to contain special chemicals which, among other things, arrest the growth of other plants unlucky enough to grow in their vicinity. These 'allelochemicals' have now been shown to inhibit the growth of tumours and of certain cancerous cells in tissue-culture; while in France it has been found that one such chemical, juglone, greenprinted in the Walnut, can arrest certain types of skin cancer. Any reader who has a Walnut tree in the garden will know the action of this alle-lochemical on the plants which do their best to grow beneath its shade. The search is now on for the healing chemicals still hidden in the Daisy for, as Shakespeare also wrote,

And this our life exempt from public haunt
Finds tongues in trees, books in the running brooks,
Sermons in stones and good in every thing.

Again and again we find throughout ancient literature references to substances produced by plants which are said to have far-reaching and strange effects on animals and humans. Pick a Dandelion and wet the bed; eat it and you certainly could, for the milky latex contains an active diuretic. Dandelion leaves make a great addition to any salad.

Lettuce, which we all now take for granted, when introduced from the wild into the Tudor diet was also rich in latex well-laced with a sedative which brought on sleep: one reason perhaps why it was a favourite of Bad King Henry VIII. Only long years of selection and breeding have turned the Lettuce into the bland basis of the starter or salad we have come to know today, hinted at in these lines by ancient Roman writer Martial:

Tell me why Lettuce, which our Grandsires last did eat,
Is now of late become, to be the first of meate.

So I went on to the Tower in search of healing plants and in the moat I found another dwarfing herb, Italian Rye, among the grasses which now line the first line of defence of those famous ramparts.

DOCKLANDS

Sad brown tufts of dead and dying plants all along my route were witness to the widespread use of new synthetic allelochemicals accurately directed, one hopes, from a spray gun. In my botanical wanderings I suffered more than a homeopathic dose of lead-free petrol, allelopathic doses of the other dearer sort, and one whiff from the not-so-distant past as an enthusiast roared by on her vintage Harley Davidson lubricated with castor oil. I wish it had been a Scott's Super Sports water-cooled, for that is the motorcycle my Dad had

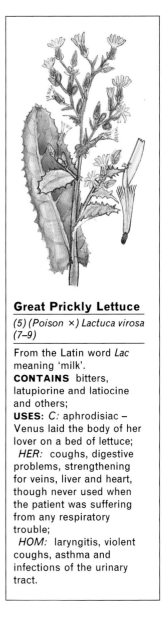

Great Prickly Lettuce
(5) (Poison ×) Lactuca virosa (7–9)

From the Latin word *Lac* meaning 'milk'.
CONTAINS bitters, latupiorine and latiocine and others;
USES: *C:* aphrodisiac – Venus laid the body of her lover on a bed of lettuce;
  HER: coughs, digestive problems, strengthening for veins, liver and heart, though never used when the patient was suffering from any respiratory trouble;
  HOM: laryngitis, violent coughs, asthma and infections of the urinary tract.

always hoped to own, but back in those days the salary of even a manager of Boots Cash Chemists did not run to such frivolities. Yet he did serve castor oil over his counter, not to lubricate bikes but to do the same to people; foul-tasting it was but a sure-fire, indeed a spectacular, purge. I was, unfortunately, one of those people who suffered the tail-end of some 300 years of what is best called 'heroic medicine', which believed in regular motions or regular purging, and there was none better to induce this than castor oil.

Introduced from tropical Asia via Egypt at least 6000 years ago, the plant was not part of British medical practice until the eighteenth century, when the art of cold-pressing was learnt. This removed the oil from the seeds but left a drastic poison, ricinine, behind.

Gerard certainly did not use castor oil but he could well lay claim to being one of the first Londoners to grow the Potato. Introduced from South America it is, along with the Tomato which came by the same route, a member of the Deadly Nightshade Family. It is hard to imagine the evolution either of 'fast food' or of our modern diet without these two denizens of the New World so perhaps a few words from Gerard concerning these staples of Macdonalds, Harry Ramsdens and the Pizza Parlour would not come amiss.

Castor Oil Plant

(Poison ××××) Ricinus communis (7–8)

Ricinus, Latin for 'a tick' – an external parasite which the strange seed resembles.
CONTAINS fatty oils, sugar, resins and the toxic alkaloid ricinin;
USES: lamp oil;
HER: gentle purgative once the alkaloid has been removed. The scaly seed must never be eaten; some people find the plant toxic in an enclosed space.

Potato

(Poison ×××) Solanum tuberosum (6–7)

CONTAINS a number of alkaloids, up to 1 per cent in the fruit, very little in the tuber except around the buds (eyes) when exposed to light. Although the tuber contains vitamins B1, B2, B6, C and PP (B3), they are destroyed by cooking.
USES: culinary;
HER: juice of the tuber is used as an antacid and anti-cramp.

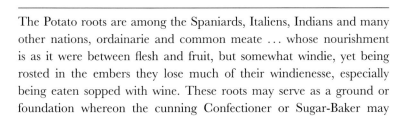

The Potato roots are among the Spaniards, Italiens, Indians and many other nations, ordainarie and common meate … whose nourishment is as it were between flesh and fruit, but somewhat windie, yet being rosted in the embers they lose much of their windienesse, especially being eaten sopped with wine. These roots may serve as a ground or foundation whereon the cunning Confectioner or Sugar-Baker may worke and frame many comfortable delicat Conserves and restorative sweet-meates … others do serve them with prunes and so eat them, likewise others dresse them (being rosted first) with oyle vinegar, and salt, every man according to his owne taste and liking.

Shades of French fries and chips to come; I wonder how prune-flavoured crisps would go down? 'Notwithstanding however they be dressed they comfort, nourish and strengthen the bodie.'

Tomatoes, or Apples-of-Love as they were then known, were first regarded as an aphrodisiac by the courtiers and courtesans who needed and could afford such luxuries. Yet Gerard says,

In Spaine and those hot regions they used to eate the Apples prepared and boyled with peper, salt and oyle, but they yeeld very little nourishment to the body and the same naught and corrupt. Likewise do they eate the Apples with oyle, vinegre and pepper mixed together for sauce to their meate even as we in those cold countries doe Mustard.

Luck was with me, I found all three – Castor Oil Plant, Potato and Tomato – growing wild in still-forgotten corners of Docklands, along with Common Fumitory and Canary-Grass – all this not far from Canary Wharf which now overshadows the City in many ways. This grass, at least, was a reminder of the once sustainable life of the estuary which, in the old days, supplied the people of London with a goodly amount of shellfish, including succulent oysters which were then so common that they were the food of the poor. Common Fumitory is as its name suggests – a common plant from the garden, especially on rich soil where it springs from the ground as if by magic, and with a juice that causes your eyes to water, like smoke, hence its Latin name *Fumaria*. Pull it up by the root and a smell like the fumes of nitric acid pervades the air.

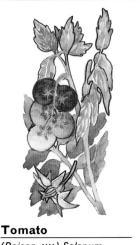

Tomato

(Poison ××) Solanum lycopersicum (6–10)

CONTAINS solanine (a potent alkaloid, only a trace of which is found in the fruits, however some people are allergic to them), vitamins C and protovitamin A which helps give the colour to the fruit; **USES:** *HER/HOM:* migraines and rheumatism.

Common Fumitory

(2) Fumaria officinalis (5–10)

Fumaria is Latin for 'smoke of the earth'.
CONTAINS at least seven alkaloids, the most abundant being fumarine, glycosides and mucilages;
USES: *C:* the 'smoke' was thought to drive away evil spirits;
  HER: to stop eyelashes growing, laxative, diuretic, eczema and dermatitis.

THE CITY OF LONDON

So to Billingsgate, the traditional fish market, and to the foot of the Monument which holds a very special place in the history of healing in London. The tower was raised to commemorate the place where the first Great Fire of London was thought to have begun. A catastrophe yes, but a medical blessing in disguise, for it burned down much of the flea- and rat-infested tenements which had harboured the plague and many other woeful diseases, thus giving London a new and healthier start.

From high on top of the Monument I looked over to the dome of St Paul's, dwarfed by the new high-rises, and remembered the second Great Fire which, along with the bombing raids of the Second World War, again destroyed so much, but not the now-dwarfed cathedral. It was in those ruins, there by courtesy of Adolf Hitler, that I first became acquainted with plants such as Rosebay Willow-herb, Melilot, Evening Primrose and Buddleia; all four were introductions from abroad and all helped to cover the wounds of urban war with a patchwork of hope.

The lax sulphur-yellow flowers of Evening Primrose turned up on the London scene from North America in 1619, a prized possession of gardeners such as John Parkinson. Its virtues long went unrecognised, for only in recent times has it been found that the oil contained in its seeds can help to reduce premenstrual tension.

Melilot was grown near London by William Turner in 1548 at Syon House where he was physician to the Duke of Somerset, Edward

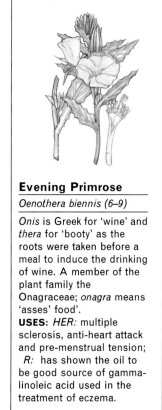

Evening Primrose

Oenothera biennis (6–9)

Onis is Greek for 'wine' and *thera* for 'booty' as the roots were taken before a meal to induce the drinking of wine. A member of the plant family the Onagraceae; *onagra* means 'asses' food'.
USES: *HER:* multiple sclerosis, anti-heart attack and pre-menstrual tension;
 R: has shown the oil to be good source of gamma-linoleic acid used in the treatment of eczema.

Melilot

(Poison ×××) Melilotus officinalis (6–9)

Wild Lote, a name given to the plant by William Turner, it is also known as King's Clover, perhaps because it took over the farms of the Tudor peasantry.
CONTAINS a glycoside melilotoside which produces coumarin on drying;
USES: *HER:* reduces bruising and so aids healing, anti-cramps, as a diuretic and for heart complaints;
 R: oral anti-coagulant used as a 'clotbuster' in treating heart attacks.

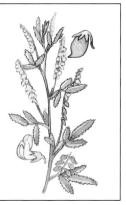

Seymour. Called King's Clover by apothecaries it was used in the then famous Melilot Plaster. This treatment was a firm favourite of Henry VIII who, like many monarchs before and after him, was a great believer in herbal healing. Henry went a lot further than most: he was interested in and indulged in the inventing, prescribing, mixing and compounding of medicines. Barbara Griggs tells us, 'His strenuous sexual life appears to have brought its own problems. "The King's Grace's oynment" was invented at St James's "to coole and dry and comfort the Member".' Among the ingredients he used were Plantain, Mallow and Sweet Violet.

Melilot was introduced into North America early this century where it was found that hay containing this plant could cause death in cattle. Their blood would not clot and so they bled to death. The active element was found to be dicoumarol, one of the chemicals causing that scent of new-mown hay. This is how the array of oral clot-busters came into being for treating heart attacks. One of them, a synthetic called warfarin, soon became one of the most effective rat poisons.

The only plant I found growing near Pudding Lane was Buddleia, which must now rank as one of London's commonest plants, along with Oxford Ragwort. Capital records to date list no medicinal properties for Buddleia but the therapeutic value of the butterflies which visit its many flowers, yes even in the city, must do wonders for all those new yuppie post-prandial tensions. One can only wonder what the 'Doctrine of Signatures' would have made of its semi-erect mauve-blue flowering spikes. Along with Salep houses it could yet replace the sordid sex shops which now serve tired business people and tourists alike.

A little bit of kerb-crawling on my part revealed a beautiful specimen in full flower complete with a Red Admiral feeding upon it. I hoped that the common Nettle was growing nearby because, although this butterfly can sip nectar from many different plants, it can only complete its life-cycle by laying its eggs on Nettles. In the country the Nettle was called Naughty Man's Plaything and Hokey Pokey, while it was sold in the streets of London to the cry of, 'Nettles with tender shoots to cleanse the blood, come buy my fresh Nettles.'

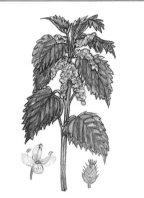

Stinging Nettle

Urtica dioica (6–10)

The word nettle comes from the fact that its stems contain strong fibre used in the manufacture of nets. When woven into cloth and washed it becomes as smooth as silk. Marama, an Irish donkey in legend, would not eat or trample nettles, but in late autumn would gently tug at the stems to get the food stored in the underground runners.

CONTAINS irritant, vitamins, protein, silica, iron and sodium;

USES: fibres, dyes (green from leaves, yellow from the root), tea, beer, wine;

C: antidote for most poisons and for some snakebite;

HER: gout, asthma, rubbing the body with fresh leaves treated hypothermia and also alleviated the pain of rheumatism, diuretic and hair restorer;

HOM: to cure its own sting, eczema and menstrual bleeding.

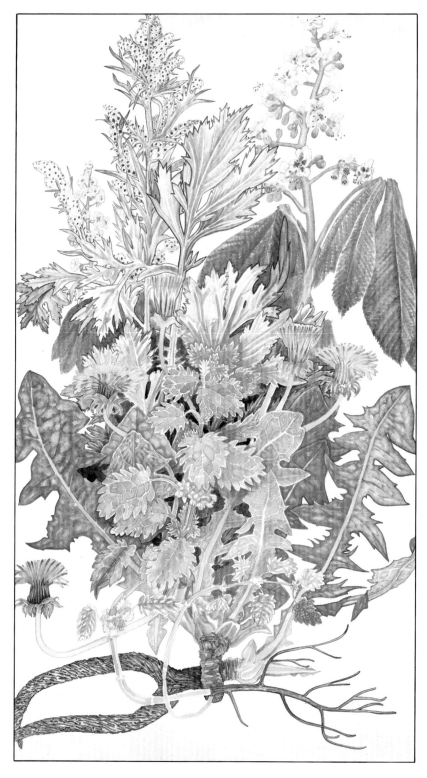

In the City of London

1 Dandelion, *Taraxacum officinale*
2 Mugwort, *Artemisia vulgaris*
3 Horse-chestnut, *Aesculus hippocastanum*
4 Small Nettle, *Urtica urens*

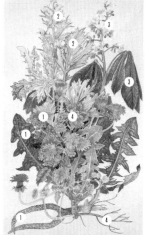

THE EMBANKMENT

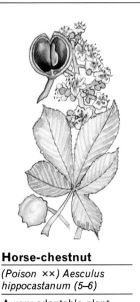

On the way to Lambeth where my grandfather, a tanner by trade and Baptist lay-preacher by conversion, was married, I passed down Huggin Hill where, in a corner still left after recent excavations, I found a patch of Nettles; enough to satisfy a small brood of 'midshipmen' caterpillars, doomed to extinction by concrete in the not too far distant future.

Horse-chestnut was also not difficult to find because it has been a favourite with landscape architects since it was introduced to this country in the fifteenth century. Today, sandwiched between mirror-glass buildings, it provides avenues stretching away into the nadirs of infinity, all for the price of two trees. It was first mentioned by the Italian physician Andrea Mathioli who used extracts of the bark to cure malaria and other intermittent fevers which were then on the rampage through the capitals of Europe. John Parkinson reported that it could cure broken-winded horses, and modern research has shown that decoctions of the bark have a specific action on blood circulation through the capillaries of the lower bowel in humans. Both bark and large shining seeds, for it is botanically incorrect to call them nuts, are used in herbal baths and it appears they have been ever since herbal baths were invented.

The Romans who bathed in the famous baths at Huggin Hill would not have been able to enjoy the luxury of the soothing Horse-chestnut and games of conkers. Possibly it was the only game in which they did not indulge, for so shocked was the Emperor Hadrian at the goings-on in this particular establishment that he banned mixed bathing throughout the Roman Empire.

Another tree I found in abundance all along my route was one that would have seemed familiar to the Romans, at least back home, the Plane. The more knowledgeable amongst them would have known that it was under such a tree on the island of Kos that the Hippocratical School of ethical medicine had had its origins. They would, however, have been wrong, for the London Plane is a more recent addition to the flora of Europe, a hybrid between the Oriental Plane, which does grow on the island of Kos, and another Plane introduced from the New World.

Horse-chestnut

(Poison ××) Aesculus hippocastanum (5–6)

A very adaptable plant which will grow on any soil and under a range of climatic conditions. Bees love it and honey produced in areas dominated by Oil-seed Rape often contains some of its virtue, for the bees flock to the trees for a change of diet.
CONTAINS soaps, tannins, a glycoside which gives a coumarin and flavones.
USES: ornamental tree;
  C: ague;
  HER: haemorrhoids and varicose veins, diuretic, herbal baths; Bach;
  R: increases the rate of circulation of the blood, having a special action on the lower bowel and so used in cases of enteritis and malfunction of the prostate.

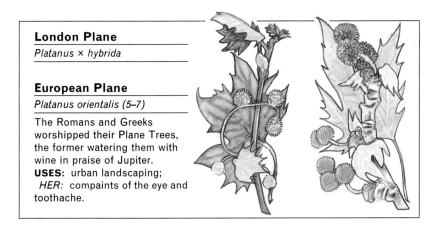

London Plane

Platanus × hybrida

European Plane

Platanus orientalis (5–7)

The Romans and Greeks worshipped their Plane Trees, the former watering them with wine in praise of Jupiter.
USES: urban landscaping;
 HER: compaints of the eye and toothache.

THE LAMBETH WALK

Lambeth was home to John and John Tradescant, a father-and-son team, gardeners to King Charles II and plant hunters and importers *par excellence*. The younger John travelled widely through the expanding colonies of North America, returning home with many plants which he grew, multiplied and sold at the so-called Lambeth Ark; part museum, part garden centre. One plant which bears their name is perhaps the first plant name most people learn to say in Latin, *Tradescantia virginiana*. The Tradescants brought this back from Virginia, a place where, unfortunately for the addicted multitudes, Tobacco – another member of the Deadly Nightshade Family – also does so well.

St Mary's Lambeth, the church in which my grandparents were married, is well worth a visit. Although it stands by the gate of the Archbishop of Canterbury's London residence, it was deemed to be redundant – well I suppose he doesn't need to go to his local church – and doomed to high-rise development. Saved by the Tradescant Trust, it is now a fitting memorial to the two Johns as it has been recycled as London's own Museum of Gardening. The churchyard comes complete with a garden of the correct period and the grave of one William Bligh of *Bounty* fame. Lest we forget, the infamous mutiny took place while the ship was on a voyage carrying plants of the Bread Fruit from the Old World to the New. These were going to be planted to feed the slaves who were then making a similar journey but under even more abominable conditions than the crew of the *Bounty*.

Among many other plants, the Tradescants grew specimens of the Oriental Plane alongside a very similar tree they had brought back from America. There, or in the Botanic Gardens in Oxford with which they regularly swapped plants, the two trees found themselves within pollinating distance after millions of years in genetic isolation. The consummation of this postponed transatlantic marriage produced a new species, the London Plane, endemic to Britain but not for long. It thrived so well in its urban setting and its trunk always looked clean and dappled with light, thanks to its flaking bark, that it was soon planted far and wide across the cities of the world. Some of the oldest are in Berkeley Square, which has a branch of Culpeper's on one corner, still carrying on the herbal traditions of all our pasts.

Doing the Lambeth walkabout as my grandparents had done before me, I chanced upon three other five-star plants, Mugwort, Feverfew and Opium Poppy, all tucked away behind the forecourt of a petrol station.

Mugwort, like all plants named after Artemis, the Roman name for the Greek Goddess Diana, is dangerous in large doses. Apuleius wrote, 'Of all those worts that we name Artemisia, it is said that Diana did find them and delivered their powers of leechdom to Cheiron the Centaur.' Long used in medicine and in alcoholic drinks as a stimulant, it is now banned in most countries because that stimulant is now known to affect the brain; so much so that the imbibing of too much absinthe caused madness and premature death in many people. Mixed with myrrh, it was used as a pessary to speed birth and ease the

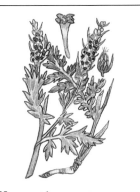

Mugwort

(23) (Poison ××) Artemisia vulgaris (8–10)

A very common plant of disturbed places and one of the first to return to Britain after the Ice Age. **CONTAINS** essential oils which include cuneol, resins and bitters; **USES:** aperitif;
 C: to stimulate the bile and get rid of worms;
 HER: aperitif, to regulate periods;
 HOM: epilepsy, and to get rid of the worm *Oxyuris*. In Chinese medicine it is the herb burned in moxibustion treatment.

passing of the placenta; while the *Polyolbion*, written by Michael Drayton in 1622, recommends, 'The belly hurt by birth, by Mugwort to make it sound.'

Feverfew, another plant with a bitter absinthe-like taste, was frequently mixed with wine and honey as a cure

Feverfew

(10) (Poison ×) Chrysanthemum parthenium (6–8)

Legend has it that this herb was used to cure a man who fell during the building of the Parthenon. It is certainly always to hand on building sites and ruins alike.
CONTAINS an essential oil with camphor, terpenes and bitters;
USES: against clothes moths;
 C: agues and other fevers. Boiled with nutmeg and mace in white wine to ease childbirth, and regulate and calm menstrual pains;
 HER/HOM: neuralgia, migraines, nervous sickness and to reduce fevers.

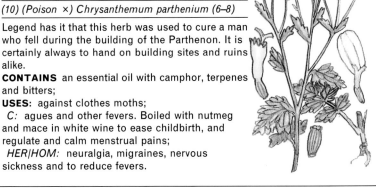

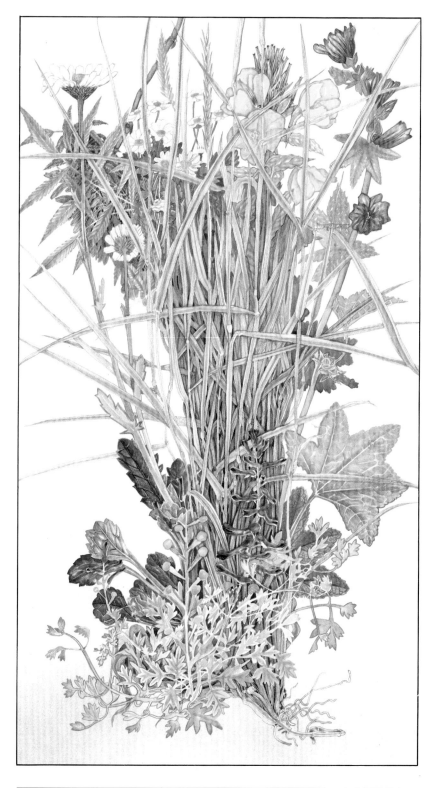

The Embankment en route to Lambeth

1 Common Fumitory, *Fumaria officinalis*
2 Dog-daisy, *Chrysanthemum leucanthemum*
3 Ash, *Fraxinus excelsior*
4 Couch-grass, *Agropyron repens*
5 Evening Primrose, *Oenothera biennis*
6 Common Mallow, *Malva sylvestris*
7 Feverfew, *Chrysanthemum parthenium*

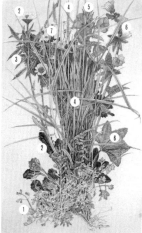

for 'them that are giddie in the head' and those 'as be melancholike' according to Gerard. Recent revelations about it being a cure for migraine are borne out by some but derided by others. For those long-suffering with this complaint, which is enough to make the happiest of us melancholy, all I can advise is to give it a try, under supervision, but remember the warning of Artemis.

The Opium Poppy has long provided medicine with its best pain-killing drug, morphine, which was openly on sale and even an ingredient of babies' gripe-water until early this century. No wonder people slept well; and surely some became addicted to this, to hemp, tobacco, alcohol or one of the other opiates used to relieve the boredom of urban living.

Opium is one of the plant kingdom's answers to pain, mimicking the effects of our own inbuilt pain-killers, the endorphins which are produced deep in the oldest part of our brains and are always there on demand. Which came first, the opiates homeopathed on the winds that blow everyone so much good or the deep endorphins there to be called upon as the need arose, killing pain and speeding our bodies into their natural cycle of recovery – the very basis of homeopathic theory and practice?

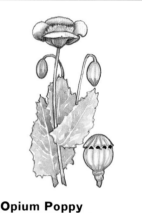

Opium Poppy

(Poison ××××) Papaver somniferum (6–8)

The seeds of the Opium Poppy contain an innocuous oil used in cooking, the rest of the plant is well laced with a milky latex which contains some at least of twenty-five nasty alkaloids. These include morphine, narcotine and codeine. The plant has been used throughout medical history to relieve pain.

CHELSEA AND ITS PHYSIC GARDEN

My granny had two addictions: Church, twice every Sunday; and lozenges compounded of Linseed, Liquorice and Chlorodyne – two mild purges and one stopper-upper, a trinity of helpful chemicals, the last of which could become addictive.

Liquorice root and the rubbery black extract going under the Italian name of Solazzi can still be bought to this day in well-stocked chemists' shops. Used for millennia in China and Egypt, Dioscorides recommended it for hoarseness and heartburn, and Theophrastus to combat cramp caused by stomach ulcers. Modern research is showing how right they were because included in its woody root is a non-fattening sweetener, much stronger than sugar, and also an anti-inflammatory, glycyrrhizic acid, great for gastric ulcers.

Linseed comes from Flax and, although I could find none growing

Liquorice

(1) Glycyrrhiza glabra (6–7)

CONTAINS glycyrrhizine fifty to sixty times as sweet as sugar, minerals, flavones and several hormones akin to our oestrogens.
USES: sweetmeats;
  C/HER: sore throats and heartburn, dropsy and dressing wounds, thirst quencher and to combat cramps caused by stomach ulcers and asthma.

wild in London, it may yet return in force because the fields of England are once again ablaze with its blue flowers, and the starlings which migrate into the city to sleep every night like to eat the seeds. *Linum usitatissimum* is a very useful plant: its seeds exude an oil, a rich source of those now all-important unsaturated fatty acids. In Gerard's own words, 'The oyle which is pressed out of the seed, is profitable for many purposes in Physicke and Surgerie.' He also adds a warning for those now true-blue new-age farmers who have added it to their high-output systems: 'Pliny saithe ... that it burneth the grounde and maketh it worser'.

> Flaxe and Oates sowing consume
> The moisture of a fertile field.
> The same worketh Poppy, whose
> Juyce a deadly sleepe doth yield.

Two warnings in one verse from a translation of a poem written by Virgil more than 2000 years ago. Flax, which also provides linen for bandages and bedclothes, was one of the main plants grown in the walled gardens around the medieval hospital of Soutra high in the borders of Scotland.

In order to find Liquorice and Flax I had to cheat and take a look in a garden, so I travelled upriver to one of my favourite spots in London. I studied botany at Chelsea Polytechnic and at lunchtimes would walk down from the King's Road, all abustle with the new promise of Mary Quant and the Temperance Seven busking on the corner, to a magic triangle close to the River Thames. There, like an elegant half-round salad sandwich, lay Chelsea Physic Garden, flanked by the Embankment, Royal Hospital Road and Swan Walk.

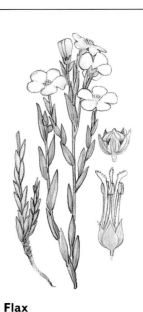

Flax

(1) Linum usitatissimum (6–7)

CONTAINS fatty oils, pectin and organic acids, vitamin F and a cyanide containing glycoside;
USES: a good source of unsaturated fatty acid oil for cooking;
  C: pain-relieving laxative;
  HER: inflammation of the digestive and urinary tracts, soothing poultices.

Founded in 1673 by the Society of Apothecaries of London, it has served the capital well, in sickness and in health. It is a place where students come to learn about plants, how to name them, how to grow them but, above all, how to use their virtues. Central to that learning are the so-called 'Order Beds' and stove-houses where the plants, drawn from all over the world, are grown in their family groups in order that we may see their similarities and their points of difference. So I shall, if I may, as I did all those years ago, indulge myself in a little bit of botany.

AN ALPHABET OF BEAUTY AND HOPE

● **Amaranthaceae** – Amaranthus Family
Provides our gardens with the highly decorative plant we call Love-lies-bleeding. Also provides us with the Grain Amaranthis, an abundant source of highly nutritious flour for the many people who are today becoming allergic to cereals in any shape or form.

● **Berberidaceae** – Barberry Family
Provides our gardens with those wonderful spring flowers and fruitful hedges made of Barberry and, thanks to the wisdom of the North American Indians, the virtues of the May Apples. Used to treat skin growths, warts and the like, although too toxic for internal use. Semi-synthetic derivatives are now used to treat cancer of the lung, kidney and testis.

● **Compositae** – Daisy Family
Our gardens abound with many sorts of Daisies and Sunflowers. Chinese Mugwort has been used in its homeland as a traditional cure for malaria for thousands of years. Artemesin or *quinghasai* as the locals call it, is now used in its pure form to treat the dreaded cerebral malaria which has become resistant to modern synthetic drugs.

● **Dioscoreaceae** – Yam Family
The family which has given the world a method of synthesising the human sex hormone progesterone, and so the first oral contraceptive: a breakthrough of immense value in an overcrowded world.

● **Ephedraceae** – Ephedra Family

A strange plant, which is grown by keen gardeners as a point of interest for it is a very primitive member of the flower-bearers, having some attributes of the cone-bearing plants. Thanks again to the wisdom of Chinese traditional medicine, its active element, ephedrine, became available to a sneezing world. A decongestant used to treat hay-fever and colds and to prevent trauma of the eardrum, it is now synthesised in vast amounts.

● **Flacourtiaceae** – Chaulmoogra Family

Although it provides no plants for our gardens, for many years an oil extracted from the Chaulmoogra tree, which grows in the forests of Burma, was the only real cure for leprosy.

● **Geraniaceae** – Geranium Family

What would our gardens be like without the Pelargoniums and Geraniums? Please get them right: the latter have regular flowers, which means that you can cut them in half in any direction and the two halves would be exactly the same. Take a look at yours and make quite sure. The oils from many members of the family are used in perfumes and aromatherapy.

● **Hamamelidaceae** – Witch Hazel Family

Witch Hazel was used by North American Indians as a soothing astringent for burns, wounds and piles; and so too was in Britain, after it had added its distinctive perfume and winter colour to our gardens.

● **Iridaceae** – Iris Family

Apart from the Freesias, Crocuses, Gladioli, Sisyrinchiums and Irises of our gardens, the family provides us with Saffron, a pigment used both in cooking and in medicines, and the infamous Syrup of Squills, a purge of heroic medicine best forgotten.

● **Juglandaceae** – Walnut Family

Walnuts and Pecans both look like a tiny human brain and so, thanks to the 'Doctrine of Signatures', were used to treat various diseases of that all-important organ. Only more recently has its dwarfing allelopathic nature been discovered. Pickled Walnuts and Pecan pie are firm favourites of mine.

● **Krameriaceae** – Krameria Family
The root of the Ratany, a perennial shrub from South America, is one of the most powerful astringents both for internal and external use.

● **Loganiaceae** – Buddleia Family
A regular chemist's shop of trees, shrubs and climbers from the forests of the tropics and sub-tropics. This family has given us curare, which paralyses the endings of our motor nerve-cells, so causing paralysis of the whole body; *Nux vomica* with strychnine-like properties; and Yellow Jessamine, still used in China and Japan to treat migraine and certain very painful forms of neuralgia.

● **Menispermaceae** – 'Open-heart Surgery Family'
A vine from the tropical rainforests of South America provided the local Indians with a paralysing poison with which to tip their arrow-heads. Modern medicine now uses the alkaloid it contains, tuboc-urarine, to relax the muscles of the heart in open-heart surgery.

● **Nymphaeaceae** – Water-lily Family
What would our rivers, streams and garden ponds be like without the Water-lilies, potent or impotent?

● **Oleaceae** – Olive Family
The Chelsea Physic Garden houses the oldest and largest Olive tree in Britain; and the whole world now benefits from the slightly laxative oil used since Egyptian times in cooking and medicine.

● **Piperaceae** – Pepper Family
When Pepper was first introduced into Europe from India, along what became known as the Spice Routes, it was of great value. Alaric, who conquered Rome in AD 408, demanded a ton of Pepper as part of the ransom – around £30 million in present-day terms. A stimulant, carminative and diuretic, today we take its virtues for granted.

● **Quinnaceae** – Quinna Family
A family still confined to the tropical forests of South America and the West Indies. We can only hope that its virtues are discovered before all the forests are destroyed.

● **Rutaceae** – Rue Family
Rue is a garden herb without equal: as a general stimulant and pick-you-up there is none better. A pleasant way to take it is in one of the great aperitifs of Italy, *Grappa-Ruta*. Pilocarpine comes from the Jaborandi of South America, it is a good remedy for acute glaucoma.

● **Scrophulariaceae** – Foxglove Family
Foxgloves in the garden, there for the bees, always reminding us of the crucially important work of William Withering.

● **Theaceae** – Tea Family
A nice cuppa, containing theophylline which, apart from doing us good in its pure and now synthetic forms, is used to reduce excess blood formation in kidney-transplant patients.

● **Umbelliferae** – Carrot Family
Caraway, Coriander, Dill and Fennel, what would our cuisine and our kitchen gardens be like without these plants?

Five thousand years before the hole in the ozone layer was discovered, the men who led the camel trains across the deserts of North Africa ate the roots of the Bullwort, *Ammi majus*, to protect themselves from sunburn. It is now known to contain methoxsalen, a chemical currently used to treat certain malignancies of the skin. It is also used with ultraviolet therapy in the treatment of psoriasis and vitiligo.

A closely-related species, the Khella, *Ammi visnaga*, was taken by a medical technician for renal colic, again following the directives of Egyptian medicine, and it relieved his heart condition, angina. That was in 1945 and subsequent research led to the synthesis of three new drugs: nifedipine used for angina and hypertension, amiodarone for abnormal beating of the heart, and 'Intal' for asthma.

What other wonders await discovery in the world of the Carrot?

● **Valerianaceae** – Valerian Family
The Common Valerian has long been used in the treatment of the heart, later it was used with success for psychoneuroses, while recent research on its essential oils reveal a family of promising sedatives.

● **Winteraceae** – Winter's Bark Family
Members of this family from the southern hemisphere can be grown

in frost-free areas of our gardens. Well worth the effort too, for it is one of the most primitive of all the flowering plants. Known to be an antiscorbutic, so useful for treating scurvy, what other virtues await discovery in this part of the basic genetic stock of all our flowers?

● **Xanthorrhoeaceae** – Grass Tree Family
Striking plants of the song lines of the Australian Aborigines. Many of the plants produce gums used in aboriginal medicine, all await research to elucidate their healing virtues.

● – Yucca Flower Family
There are no plant families which begin with Y in Latin, for there is no such letter in that alphabet. Yucca has long been used by the Indian people of South West USA for the treatment of arthritis and rheumatism.

● **Zingiberaceae** – Ginger Family
Ginger, which followed Pepper and all the others along the spice routes from the East, soon became part of many prescriptions. Modern research using double-blind trials on two randomly-selected and treated groups of patients, neither the patients nor the researchers knowing who is having which treatment, have come up with some fascinating results. A substance extracted from ginger root has been shown to be far superior to long-established synthetic antihistamines in preventing motion sickness. As the Chelsea Physic Garden's introductory leaflet says, 'A surprising finding which demonstrates the importance of the proper scientific testing of old herbal remedies.'

To date, only about 1 per cent of all the flowering plants growing in the world have been put to modern test. Thanks to work at places such as Chelsea Physic Garden, the Royal Botanic Gardens at Kew, and other botanic gardens and universities across the world, the knowledge of old herbal remedies is now being used as a key to unlock the hidden treasure-chest of healing virtues.

Many of the plants listed in this book may be grown in your local parks, your garden or even a window-box. It will be worth doing this for then you will have a wildlife garden providing you with the benefit, not only of the beauty, but also of their 'homeopathic' presence; an enfleurage of our pasts and hope for all our futures.

The Tree of Life

*W*hen St Augustine came to Britain in the sixth century to preach Christianity he was told to purify but not to destroy the temples of pagan worship.

There seems little doubt that the evergreen Yew was a sacred tree, not only to the Druids but also to the Celtic stock which moved north-west across Europe in the warming post-Ice Age days. In landscapes which were mainly covered with deciduous trees, Yews would have been easy to pick out in the winter and, with their crop of coral-red berries, they certainly looked out of place: exotic, even tropical. Very early on, the trial and error process of discovery must have had its fatalities both from animals eating the leaves and people the fruits, for although the pink flesh is wholesome, containing mucilages and sugar, the hard seed contains the drastic poison alkaloid called taxine. Yew also provided wood for the shafts of spears and for longbows. The generic name comes from *Taxus*, meaning arrow. Yew was thus a plant to be feared, yet one to be revered as the Tree of Life for they live to a gnarled old age.

Pliny wrote, 'It is unpleasant and fearful to look upon, as a cursed tree, without any liquid substance at all.' Gerard may have scoffed at the old belief concerning the danger of resting beneath its shade but we know that its poisons do affect the brain, and in a warm country the dark heat-absorbing foliage might release too much of a complex of substances.

Two sets of current modern research hold the tree in high esteem. One is by an amateur, Allen Meredith, who has spent much of his life studying the Yew trees of our churchyards. By collecting pieces of wood which has fallen within their hollow trunks and counting the annual rings he has constructed a growth-curve for the trees. Now,

simply by measuring the girth of the trunk 1.5 metres (5 feet) above
the ground, it is possible to guestimate the age of a tree. Cross-
referencing his growth-curve with known planting dates and other
information gleaned from literature, Alan has come up with the fact
that many of the oldest Yews are found on the north, the dark side,
of churches and they all pre-date Christianity. Our oldest, which in
1771 had a girth of nearly 20 metres (65 feet) and could be an
incredible, unbelievable, 9000 years old, is at Fortingall in Perthshire
at the centre, or at least the centre of gravity, of what we now call
Scotland. Before you say ridiculous, cut out a map of Scotland, stick
a pin through, spin, and see for yourself. Coincidence or *Axis Mundi?*
Here, the story becomes mixed up with legends of Pontius Pilate,
whose father served in the Roman legions at Fortingall; and also with
more ancient worship because ritual pagan fires are said to have been
lit within this tree destroying any hard-core evidence of its age.
Whatever the final outcome of Allen's work, it is clear that the Yew
has long been a sacred tree.

Far away from Scotland on the Pacific coast of America there is
another type of Yew tree, an understorey plant in the greatest
rainforests of the Earth. These temperate forests stretch from northern
California through Oregon to Washington and on up into Canada.
They are dominated by enormous trees, such as the Douglas fir and
Western Hemlock, and they have twice the standing crop of timber
of any of their tropical cousins. It is for this reason and those timbers
that 87 per cent of all these forests in the USA have already been
destroyed by logging. The Pacific Yew found within the forests was
looked upon as a useless tree and was usually burned on the spot.

Almost too late, researchers found the Pacific Yew to contain a
substance called taxol which appears to give hope to people suffering
from certain types of cancer. In 1962 a scientist working at the National
Cancer Institute collected samples of the tree. Five years later, taxol
had been isolated and named. The discovery was then sat on for
twenty years until pressure from groups of lobbying patients flushed
the story out into the light of the cancer-ridden late 1980s. Soon
everyone was clamouring to get in on the taxol trials. When you are
dying or when you know someone who is dying of that dreaded
terminal disease in all its malignant forms, any chink in the consulting-

room door becomes a gateway of hope. (In America one man was found at night wandering around a university campus in search of taxol for his dying mother.)

When I was young, death from disease was a more everyday matter – pneumonia, diphtheria, scarlet fever, tuberculosis and polio. Many of these have been, at least in the rich countries, relegated to 'dread things of the past', thanks to better nutrition and hygiene, and to vaccination and the more recent magic bullets of twentieth-century medicine. Today, the main killers are the motor car, tobacco, heart attacks and cancer, the last taking pride of place in what is pre-dominantly a geriatric population. Three-score years and ten have run to more like three-score years and fifteen in the case of men and four-score plus for women in the developed world. As the body ages, its defence and control systems weaken and carcinogens find an easier prey. No wonder every decade demands new hope of a wonder cancer cure.

For years, conservationists had been trying to save those western Pacific forests from further destruction by the logging companies. One of their aims was to get the Northern Spotted Owl classified as an endangered species, for that would have forced the government to protect the last 10 per cent of their habitat. The Pacific Yew suddenly entered the argument, but on both sides. Save the forest and you save the potentially life-giving Yews. But, from the other side, we must log what's left of the forest to get at the Yews. Commonsense never has prevailed in such situations but at least the scientists realised that it would take the sacrifice of three mature Yews to provide one patient with a course of treatment; and Yews are a finite resource. If only the logging industry had helped to regrow the forest in the past and built a sustainable industry then livelihoods and lives would now be at less risk. The dilemma is still there: the more research that is done the better the drug appears to be, with remission rates reported of between 30 and 35 per cent in trials of over 200 patients suffering from ovarian cancer; initial studies of women with advanced breast cancer are also showing promising results. Time ticks away, many die, many more live in hope. What is now needed is more, lots more of the drug to be used in more widespread clinical tests.

In France scientists have discovered a method for partial synthesis of a compound obtained from the needles of the European Yew to produce a drug, Taxoterg, which was patented in 1986. It is more water-soluble than its competitor Taxol and so may not suffer from the same side-effects of administration.

The race is on, with many companies and universities entering the field for Laureates and other less noble, yet equally glistering prizes.

Work in Britain is now using a sustainable resource, the clippings from the Yew hedge maze at Longleat in Wiltshire, to provide the raw material for their research. Dr Jenkins of Leicester University commented in 1992 that he 'hopes to produce a synthetic form of taxinine soon, and within five years a total synthesis of taxol'. He also hopes 'to discover other important taxol-mimicking compounds along the way'.

The genus *Taxus* promises an entirely new armoury in the fight against the final killer, cancer; not wonder-drugs in the real sense of the word but each advance is a great step of hope for the one in five of us who are now likely to die from the disease.

The Tree of Death, which has stood for so long spreading its evergreen welcome at the churchyard gate, may once again become the Tree of Life.

Yew

(Poison ××××) – Taxus baccata*

Once worshipped as 'The Tree of Life' probably because of its longevity.
CONTAINS several very poisonous alkaloids including taxine and ephedrine, glycosides and pigments.
USES: worship, arrow poison, witchcraft.
 HER: medicine, heart problems.
 HOM: medicine, tincture for liver and kidney complaints and for rheumatism and arthritis.
 R: anti-cancer.

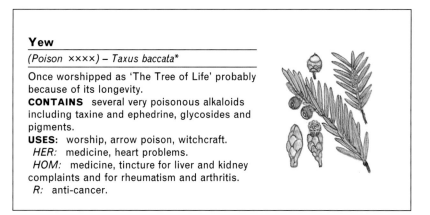

(*See page 171.)

APPENDIX I

A little bit of natural history

*L*ong before people began recording history in artefact, manu-script or books, fresh air was doing the job on a massive scale. Wherever geological deposits, rock, sediment and especially peat accumulated, part of the annual rain of pollen, spores, dust and even the organic chemicals in the air became preserved, forming a detailed record of all our pasts.

We first turn to the pollen record held fast mainly in our peatlands to discover how the natural pharmacy of Britain came into existence.

12,000 Years BP (Before Present) – The Ice Age draws to a temporary close

For the previous 35,000 years much of Britain had been covered with great sheets of ice or had been affected by permafrost, leaving the landscape littered with shattered rock, gravels, sands and silts. It was an inhospitable place, almost devoid of life but full of mineral promise.

11,000 BP – The Late Glacial Period

As the climate improved, the process of colonisation began. Plants and animals migrated in from the continent of Europe to which the British Isles were then joined. The first plants able to make themselves at home were the arctic and alpine varieties which could tolerate the intensely cold conditions. Plants such as Dwarf Juniper, Willow and Birch dominated the open tundra vegetation.

10,000 BP – The Boreal Period begins

Other larger trees including Downy and Silver Birch, Pine, Hazel, Rowan and several Willows had joined the stream of immigrants. Park tundra with clumps of trees dominated the southern lowlands and bands of Early Stone

Age (Palaeolithic) People followed the influx of plants, hunting herds of grazing and browsing animals which included reindeer, elk and even mammoth.

9000 BP

The great Boreal Forest was spreading, with Oaks, Elms and Alders making their presence felt. Deep forest soils were forming, held fast by the root systems of perennial plants. The healing process, which would eventually cover the landscape with a mantle of living forest, was in full swing.

8000 BP

By the end of the Boreal Period mixed broadleaf woodland covered the lowland of England and Wales, while Birch and Pine still dominated Scotland. The arctic, alpine and other plants of open ground were in retreat, surviving only on mountain tops, river cliffs, rocky outcrops and the like.

7000 BP – The Atlantic Period

The Earth's temperature rose to a post-glacial high, about 2.5°C warmer than it is today, and the climate of Britain also got wetter. Lime, Holly and Ash became important components of the forest while Birch and Pine were less abundant except in north and central Scotland.

The wetter weather stimulated the spread of acid peat which rapidly covered large areas of lowland wetlands with raised bogs. Blanket bogs also began to spread in the north and west. These acid peatlands were dominated by plants such as Bog Mosses and Cottons, Heathers and Heaths. As the peat grew, the greenhouse gas (carbon dioxide) was locked up out of the atmosphere, 'cooling the fever of the Earth', one is tempted to say.

6000 BP – Britain becomes a group of islands

Thanks to the continued melting of the ice sheets, both the English and Irish Channels became filled with water, flooding all the land bridges which had also been covered with Boreal Forest. At this time most of the land mass was covered with mixed deciduous forest. Only the tops of the highest mountains, steep cliffs, dunes and rock outcrops were free from the influence of forest and peat. Deer, wolves and wild oxen lived in the forest and ranged across the open wetlands, followed by an increasing population of Middle Stone Age (Mesolithic) People.

5000 BP

The end of the Atlantic Period was marked right across Europe by a dramatic reduction in the importance of Elm. Whether these mighty trees fell foul of some widespread disease, as they have in more recent times, or whether the polished axes of the People of the New Stone Age (Neolithic) cultures allowed massive forest clearance, we do not know. Elm leaves are very nutritious and were certainly fed to the cattle which were then grazed on the more open ground, but the question still remains of whether there were enough itinerant farming families to cause such widespread damage. Whatever the answer, the cooler, drier Sub-Boreal Period which followed was to see the effects of people slowly but surely change the face of the British Isles.

Areas of forest on the lighter, sandy soils of the uplands were cleared, first to make way for grazing animals, then for crops. The abundance of charcoal laid down in soils, sediments and peats at that time shows that slash-and-burn agriculture was taking its now time-dishonoured toll. Woodlands there still were in plenty, enriched by Ash and in the south by two later arrivals, Beech and Hornbeam, but more and more space was being taken up by farmland. The pollen grains of cereals such as Wheat and Barley appear along with weedy species, Plantain, Dock and Wormwood. The poorer, thinner soils were soon exhausted and, as the farmers moved on, acid heathland and chalk and limestone grassland healed the eroding land. It was probably the Neolithic farmers who first developed the art and craft of coppicing. Many of the trees they felled re-sprouted from the base to produce healthy young stems, ideal for all sorts of small wood uses.

4000 BP

Most of south-east England had been cleared of forest, and spiny grazing-tolerant plants such as Gorse were increasing in abundance.

3000 BP

The Sub-Boreal Period was drawing to a close and was replaced by the wetter Sub-Atlantic, the climatic period about which we all grumble to this day. The smoke of smelters' bronze and iron was added to that of slash-and-burn as forest clearance for fuel and farming proceeded furiously. The pioneer trees, Birch, Ash, Beech and Hornbeam, rapidly took over abandoned farms, and peatlands spread once again, especially along the wetter, western Celtic fringe.

2000 BP

The Romans were on their way to mix and mingle with the half a million inhabitants of Britain, bringing with them Walnut, Sweet Chestnut, Plum and Crab Apple. They built roads which opened up the more inaccessible parts of the country to agriculture, and began the drainage of the wetlands of East Anglia which were planted with cereals to feed the increasing population.

1500 BP

The Romans had come and gone, leaving their distinctive marks across the length and breadth of Britain. The heavy soils of the lowlands were still in the main wooded, except for small patches around the iron smelters. The Anglo-Saxons who took the Romans' place had stronger and heavier ploughs and so began to clear even the rich but clayey lowland soils. Many of the upland farms were abandoned as villages, each surrounded by two or three fields divided into strips, began to re-order the landscapes.

1000 BP

It was then sixty-six years before the most famous date in English history and eighty-six years before the great Domesday survey of William the Conqueror. The survey was to show that some 35 per cent of England was under arable farming, 30 per cent pasture, 15 per cent woodland and wood pasture in which animals were grazed, 1 per cent meadow (grassland cut for hay), the remaining 19 per cent was mountain, moorland, heath and houses and their gardens. The Norman kings enjoyed hunting and so large areas were set aside as royal game reserves under forest law. Nevertheless, overgrazing by cattle, sheep and pigs made the boundaries between these categories of land use a little hazy. The Normans brought rabbits with them as a convenient source of meat and fur, and as the population of these furry fiends grew and grew the chance of woodland regeneration diminished. Large areas of the fenlands were inundated by the sea flooding croplands and revitalising wetland growth.

800 BP

Monasteries were founded all around the country, often in remote places. Sheep joined the rabbits in preventing woodland regeneration, and grassland spread across the uplands of England, Wales and southern Scotland.

600 BP

The wetlands of eastern England were progressively drained and the fenlands were grazed by large herds of cattle and flocks of sheep. Woodland products were in great demand for the building of windmills, houses, churches, cathedrals and ships, especially during Tudor times.

The Stuart period saw a shortage of timber and timber products, so much so that advice was sought from the members of the newly-formed Royal Society. This advice culminated in the publication in 1664 of a 'Discourse of Forest Trees and the Propagation of Timber', known as John Evelyn's *Sylva*. Sycamore was introduced to Britain around this time.

300 BP

Little remained of the natural vegetation of the British Isles, most of which was now both people-made and people-managed. Further change came on apace with the Enclosure Act of 1750, which meant the open fields of the past were enclosed by hedges and walls. Likewise, large areas of heaths, moorlands and grassland were enclosed, improved and brought under cultivation. European Larch, Norway Spruce and Silver Fir were added to the increasing areas of plantation, which also included Oak, Ash, Beech and Pine, the latter two species often planted way beyond their natural range.

The First World War accelerated the need for home-grown timber and 1919 saw the establishment of the Forestry Commission.

The low input/low output cropping of the nineteenth century, which included self-fertilising water-meadows and crop rotation with periods of the land lying fallow as important parts of the rural economy, was slowly swept away.

50 BP

After the Second World War the change became catastrophic. During the last fifty years 97 per cent of our lowland, neutral grassland and flower-rich hay meadows, 45 per cent of what was left of our ancient and coppice woodlands, 40 per cent of lowland heaths, 80 per cent of lowland chalk and limestone grassland have all been replaced by high input/high output agriculture or plantation, and hedgerows have been destroyed. It is mainly during this time that the growing urban population has become more and more alienated from any contact with the background of natural vegetation which had affected their evolution and their well-being over the past 12,000 years.

APPENDIX II

A potted history of herbal medicine

12,000–5000 BP (Before Present)

In the warmer parts of the world away from the main effects of the Ice Age, human society and the medicine upon which it came to depend, developed more rapidly than in Britain. At first, the knowledge and practice of herbal healing must have been developed through trial and error, and there must have been some painful and catastrophic results. No doubt the hunting people watched animals very closely and learned from them. For example, just as our pet cats and dogs will eat certain plants to make them sick, so do wild animals. If they have been bitten by a snake, chamois deer are known to graze on distasteful Spurges, which give them violent diarrhoea. Wolves appear to dig up and eat the root of Bistort for the same reason. Musk rats will coat wounds with resin that they gather from Pine trees. Today, we have some evidence that hinds eat certain species of Lily to bring themselves on heat, while some apes and monkeys browse on specific types of leaves and fruits which 'regulate' conception.

Such knowledge, once gleaned, was first passed down the family line of Wise Women, grandmother to granddaughter. Then, as chauvinism began to rule some roosts, the knowledge became entangled in the rites and wrongs of shamanistic religion with all its professional jealousies.

5000–2000 BP

In China, Shen Nung, the mythical Divine Peasant, began to write the *Pen Ts'ao* which was eventually published as the *Great Herbal* some 4600 years later. In Egypt, medical papyri were written, recording the use of more than 260 plants, while in Assyria, similar information was recorded on tablets of clay which listed some 250 drugs.

In India, the Atharavaveda was handed to Brahma some time in the second century BC; it contained much herbal lore and folk medicine. In

Israel, the Talmud and the Old Testament were written; both contain many references to health practice and some to herbal medicine. The same is true of the Koran, written by the followers of Islam. Each one gives us an insight into the wonder of these great civilisations which developed in North Africa and along the shores of the Mediterranean.

2000–1000 BP

During this period we find the first records of hospitals and convalescent homes built by Buddhist monks in Sri Lanka, 397–307 BC. A little later King Asoka reigned in India, he helped to develop law, order and medicine throughout India and Sri Lanka, 247–207 BC.

The Classical Period, 2000–1000 BP

The work in the subcontinent of India carried on and between 0 and AD 700 the *Charaka Samhita* and *Susruta Samhita* were written down. These are the main foundations of Arduveyic medicine which still serves many people well to this day.

● **Hippocrates,** said to have been born around 400 BC on Kos, now known as a Greek holiday island, probably never existed. A school of medicine which bore his name definitely did. It gave the world much herbal knowledge and the Hippocratic oath of ethical conduct. Its members were the fathers of therapeutic medicine.

● **Theophrastus,** today recognised as the 'Father of Botany', was a Greek philosopher born on the island of Lesbos around 372 BC. He died in Athens some eighty-five years later.

● **Pliny the Elder** was born in Como around AD 23 and died when Vesuvius erupted fifty-six years later. He was the 'Father of Natural History', for during his lifetime he wrote thirty-seven volumes on the subject and these included descriptions of many healing plants.

● **Dioscorides** lived during the first century AD. Born in Cilicia, he wrote an enormous tome called *Materia Medica* which listed more than 500 plants. This became the main textbook of herbal medicine for the next thousand years. He also sowed the seeds of the 'Doctrine of Signatures', the theory that suggested plants which looked like parts of the human body would help cure afflictions of those parts.

● **Galen** was born in Pergamum in Greece around AD 130 and died in Italy seventy years later. He is regarded as the 'Father of Pharmacy' and some of his Galenic prescriptions are still in use today.

The Middle Ages

● **Charlemagne,** King of the Franks and Emperor of the East, was born around AD 742 at Neustrye and died in Aachen in 814. He or his son issued a number of Acts or laws, one of which stated which plants should be grown on the Royal estates.

● **Rhazes,** certainly the most famous of Islam's physicians, was born in Rayy around AD 865 and died about sixty years later, having completed a prodigious amount of work.

● **Avicenna,** one of the most famous men of the Arab world, came to be known as the 'Prince of Physicians'. Born in AD 980, he died in Hamadan fifty-seven years later, having written the amazing *Canon of Medicine* which is still in use today.

● **Saint Hildegard,** born in Germany in 1098, spent a life of saintly service creating and developing a physic garden at the Convent of Ruppertsberg near Bingen where she died in 1179.

● **Physicians of Myddfai.** Legend has it that a farm boy successfully courted and married a lady who appeared complete with dowry out of a lake in south Wales. Later, she returned from the lake and gave her three sons a packet of herbal prescriptions which were put to good use for the next thousand years. Fortunately for generations of people in rural Wales, the story of the Lady of the Lake and the prescriptions used by the Physicians of Myddfai were written down for posterity some time in the thirteenth century.

● **The Soutra hospital.** Meanwhile, some 300 miles to the north near Soutra on the main route from England to Scotland, a large hospital was at work serving the local monastic community and the many travellers who used the road. Recent excavation has unearthed large quantities of hospital waste which, in the dedicated hands of Dr Brian Moffat and his co-workers, is revealing detailed and fascinating information about medieval medicine. Despite the fact that the Soutra hospital, one of more than a thousand then built in Britain, was situated 1100 feet above sea-level, the monks grew three very important drug plants, probably in walled gardens: Flax, Hemp and Opium Poppy. They also made use of Tormentil, a native plant which grew and still grows in abundance thereabouts.

1500–1900 The age of the herbals and heroic medicine

With the advent of printing in about 1454, the scarce manuscripts of the past, which contained handwritten details of herbs and herbal medicines, were soon put into print; so the knowledge they contained, both right and wrong, were made available to those who cared to learn to read and could afford the luxury of books.

● **Philippus Aureolus Theophrastus Bombastus von Hohenheim,** known ever since as Paracelsus, the son of a Swiss physician, was born around AD 1490 near Einsiedeln. In his youth he saw the problems caused by the effects of mercury and other poisons both on the miners employed to dig them from the ground, and on their families who worked washing and extracting them from the ores. At medical school he became a rebel, counselling wise use of all medicines and pointing out the need for correct dosage in each case. If only more people had taken notice of his pleas, many would have been saved extreme suffering, for the so-called 'Heroic Medicine' relied at the time on the use of many poisons such as mercury and antimony.

While many mainstream doctors and quacks came to rely on too frequent blood letting, ultra violent emetics and purges and small but regular doses of deadly poisons which did their patients much more harm than good others continued to work wonders with plants.

Among them were the women folk from the most humble cottage to the grandest stately home. **Gervaise Markham**'s *The English Housewife*, first published in 1615, set down much of this homespun wisdom. It ran to many editions and was a best seller throughout the century, Markham acknowledged the fact that much of the contents of the book was taken from a manuscript which had belonged to **Lady Frances Countesse Dowager of Exeter**.

The first Herbal to be printed in the English language was by **Richard Banckes**. Published in 1526 it was in essence a copy of manuscripts of the fourteenth century, linking us back to the Myddfai.

● **William Turner**'s Herbal published in parts some twenty-five years later was a much more scientific work containing many of his own observations. Turner well deserves the title of Father of English Botany.

At that time Herbals were coming off the presses thick and fast and few were thicker than that of **John Gerard**'s 1630 huge pages covered with more than half a million words, complete with the woodcut illustrations. It was first published in 1597. Although Gerard stated that it was 'principally intended for gentlewomen' and despite all its faults, mistakes and plagiarisms his *Herbal or General History of Plants* become the standard work for English students.

● **John Parkinson** was another herbalist of the Grand Tradition for he ran both a lucrative and fashionable practice and kept a Physic Garden to supply his clients' herbal needs. He linked the two and his name in *Paradisi in Sole* (Park in the Sun) published in 1629.

At that time the hierarchy of healing ran something like this. At the top were the physicians, whose formal training at the universities of Oxford and Cambridge could last 14 years. There they were steeped in the classical works and the complexities of *materia medica*. Then came the surgeons who in the absence of anaesthetics were perfecting all their many techniques at lightning speed. Then the barber surgeons who did the blood-letting and tooth extraction and finally the apothecaries who kept up the supply of animal, vegetable and mineral which went into the pills and potions.

● **Nicholas Culpeper** is without doubt the best known apothecary of all time. Herbalist, astrologer and doctor he published the first English translation of the *London Dispensatory* in 1651. Until that time it had been published only in Latin by the then all important College of Physicians. This is still in print to this day and many herbal stores still carry his name and his tradition of healing.

John was a very popular name in the healing circles of those days. **John Evelyn**, a diarist who lived from 1620 to 1706 was an expert on trees and did his best to heal the depredations of agriculture and landscape mismanagement by exhorting the nation to replant its woodlands. **John Ray**, son of the blacksmith at Black Notley in Essex, excelled at Cambridge and became the local vicar in his home village. His many books extolling all the products of God's Creation earned him the title of Father of Natural History and his *Catalogus Plantarum Angliae* published in 1670 listed the plants then known to be growing in Britain, shades of many Floras to come.

The last of the real Herbals was by **John Pechey**. Published in 1694 it contained a syntheses of the best of the old redistilled through and enriched by the ideas and knowledge of people like Culpeper and Ray.

During the Industrial Revolution things went from bad to worse. The countryside could no longer support the exploding population so more and more people were forced to live in the unhealthy conditions of the new towns. There they had no access to the traditional herbal cures of the countryside and they could not afford the prices charged by the physicians and apothecaries who were few in number and therefore in great demand.

John Wesley, 1703–1791, Methodist preacher without equal, became their champion. His little pamphlet *Primitive Physic or a Natural and Easy Method of Curing Most Diseases*, published in 1781, preached good sense and the use of cheap easily obtained plant remedies, some even from the Indians of North America.

● **William Withering**, 1741–1799, graduated in Medicine from Edinburgh University steeped in mainstream practice and malpractice. He, however, learned that many of the old herbal cures had worked well over the centuries but understood the danger of medicines made from very poisonous plants. To help solve the problem he carried out pioneer and now classic research to check the plants and regularise the preparation and dosages of the medicines.

His work led on to the great corpus of research based knowledge in which Pharmaceutical Science has its foundations. Work which formed the basis of the contents of great tomes called the *British Pharmacopoeia* and *Pharmaceutical Codex*. These are continuously updated so that they purport to contain the best knowledge and practice at the date of publication.

In Germany a brilliant linguist and chemist graduated in medicine in 1799. He found that he could bring on the symptoms of a number of fevers by dosing himself with certain herbs or herbal extracts. He therefore developed the idea of homeopathy, the use of minute amounts of herbal extracts to speed the body into the 'condition' and so into the body's natural cycle of healing. His name was **Christian Friedrich Samuel Hahnemann**.

Just as John Wesley and others had brought back good news of herbal medicine as practised by the indigenous people of North America, good news began to travel fast with the increase in transatlantic travel.

● **Samuel Thompson**, 1769–1843, the son of a poor farmer from New Hampshire in America, became a champion of herbal medicine across the world. An advocate of the traditional remedies of the North American Indians and especially of their 'steam' bath techniques of aromatherapy.

A Narrative of the Life and Medical Discoveries of Samuel Thompson, published in 1825, gives a fascinating insight to these times.

● **Albert Isaiah Coffin**, 1790–1866, was also born in America. At first a great supporter of the work of Thompson he soon went his own way popularising the cause of Botanic Medicine across the length and breadth of Britain. He found a friend and colleague in another John – **John Skelton** – a herbalist from Plymouth who learned the laws of his healing profession from his grandmother, doctress and midwife in the village of Holberton in Devon where he was born in 1806. Together they provided much needed help to the millions who crowded the industrial cityscapes of those times battling against epidemics of cholera and worse.

Together and later alone and embittered against each other and their mentor, Thompson, they spawned many local institutes like the Eclectic,

Botanic, Medical and Phrenological Institute of Derby. One member of this august body was Jesse Boot of Nottingham who left and eventually turned his considerable expertise and energies on the development of, to put it in his own words: '... new chemists shops in which a greater and better variety of pharmaceutical articles could be obtained at cheaper price'.

Boots Cash Chemists did not forsake herbal medicine, it endeavoured to provide the best of the old and the then amazing new developments of twentieth-century medicine at prices the people could afford. It was at one of the branches of this Tree of Patent Medicine that I became apprenticed to a life-long interest in plants and their powers of healing.

● **Edward Bach**, 1886–1936, was born near Birmingham of Welsh stock. He worked in his father's brass foundry before going on to medical school. After a very successful practice as a doctor and physician in fashionable London, he got more and more interested in the people whom he was treating rather than the diseases from which they were suffering. He opted out of mainstream medicine and travelled widely in Britain and especially in Wales. Settling in a cottage called Mount Vernon near Oxford, he developed his now famous Bach Flower Remedies. 'Homeopathic' doses prepared from flowers steeped in spring water and set to stand in the Oxfordshire sun, or boiled in spring water, are the basis of his herbal practice. They are prescribed to cure the patient, not the disease.

Edward Bach is perhaps the best link we have between the old and the new. The immense breakthroughs of the twentieth century both in public health, and in the understanding, treatment and apparent conquest of many once, 'killer' diseases tended to push *materia medica* derived from plants out of the medical curricula and out of favour with some. This is despite the fact that many of the techniques and modern drugs are derived from the herbal traditions of the past.

Thanks to stalwarts like **Mary Grieve** and **Hilda Leyel**, two herbal healers and gardeners who between and beyond the two world wars kept the lamp of herbal common sense burning, despite many, I would say very many ill informed decisions by successive governments of all political colours. Their book, *A Modern Herbal*, first published in 1931, has likewise put much herbal knowledge into the hands and minds of those who want to take heed of the good news of the past.

These are just a few of the names of those who have made it to the written pages of history and who have educated and inspired me to write this book. There is another much larger group to whom we all owe a huge debt of gratitude: the ordinary people who have throughout this immense passage of time continued to use their own local plants to help families and friends in health and especially in sickness.

A bibliography of the more modern works to which I have referred during my research in writing this book and the television programmes which go with it is appended below:

Bibliography

ADDISON, J. *Illustrated plantlore* Sidgwick & Jackson, 1985. op.
ARBER, A. *Herbals, their origin and evolution* Cambridge U.P., 1986
GRIGGS, B. *Green pharmacy, a history of herbal medicine.* Robert Hale, 1987. op.
GRIGSON, G. *Englishman's flora* Phoenix House, 1955. op.
LINDLEY, J. *Flora medica* Longman, Orme, Brown, Green & Longmans, 1833. op.
PRATT, A. *Flowering plants, grasses, sedges and ferns of Great Britain* Warne & Co., 1899. op.
SCHAUENBERG, P. & PARIS, F. *Guide to medicinal plants* Lutterworth Press, pbk., 1990.

Useful addresses

Health Food Stores:—
National Association of Health Food Stores (NAHS), Chamber of Commerce Building, Unit 2D, Boston Industrial Centre, Norfolk Street, Boston, Lincolnshire PE21 9HG
Tel: 0205 362626

Herbal Manufacturers:—
British Herbal Manufacturers' Association, Field House, Lye Hole Lane, Redhill, Avon BS18 7TB
Contact: Ray Hill.

Practitioners:—
Institutute of Complementary Medicine, 21 Portland Place, London W1N 3AP
National Institute of Medical Herbalists, 41 Hatherley Road, Winchester, Hampshire SO22 6RR

Homeopathic Organizations:—
The Faculty of Homeopathy, The Royal London Homeopathy Hospital, Great Ormond Street, London WC1N 3HR
The Society of Homeopaths, 2 Artizan Road, Northampton NN1 4HU
British Homeopathic Association, 27A Devonshire Street, London W1N 1RJ

Conservation Bodies:—
Royal Society for Nature Conservation, Your Local County Conservation and Wildlife Trusts, Witham Park, Waterside South, Lincoln LN5 7JR
R.S.P.B., The Lodge, Sandy, Bedfordshire SG19 2DL
Woodland Trust, Autumn Park, Dysart Road, Grantham, Lincolnshire NG31 6LL
Plant Life, c/o The British Museum of Natural History, Kensington, London SW7 5BD
Wildfowl & Wetland Trust, Slimbridge, Gloucestershire GL2 7BT

INDEX

Page numbers in *italic* refer to the illustrations